Scleroderma Coping Strategies

by

B. Bianca Podesta

Foreword by Lee S. Shapiro, M.D.

Two Harbors Press
212 3rd Avenue North, Suite 290
Minneapolis, MN 55401
612.455.2293
www.TwoHarborsPress.com

ISBN-13: 978-1-936401-18-5
LCCN: 2010941888

Distributed by Itasca Books

Cover Design by Carolyn Corse
Typeset by Wendy Arakawa

Printed in the United States of America

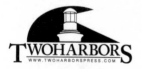

The information in this book is not intended to diagnose, treat, cure, or prevent any disease, nor has this material been evaluated by the Food and Drug Administration. All information relating to medical conditions, health issues, products, and treatments are not meant to be a substitute for the advice of your physician or other medical professional. Do not use the information in this book to diagnose or to treat yourself. Consult with your physician or medical professional before making changes to medications or doctor recommended programs of any kind.

For those who want to know more about scleroderma, and for my sister and brother patients who have inspired and encouraged this project.

If it hurts to eat, to breathe, to move, to think, to love, you may want to stop trying. Don't stop trying. Persist until you find a way, by natural means if possible, to reduce or to eliminate the pain.

CONTENTS

FOREWORD

Bianca Podesta has produced an insightful book on coping with the effects of an incurable systemic illness, using her own experience with scleroderma as a model.

Scleroderma, which means "hard skin," is an autoimmune connective tissue disease; the hardness comes from an overproduction of collagen that may occur not only in the skin but in other body tissues and organ systems. This can result in loss of function and, sometimes, loss of life. Until a cure is found, our common goal is to promote the highest degree of wellness for people living with this disease.

For a physician who specializes in the diagnosis and treatment of scleroderma, reading Podesta's journal excerpts is a sobering exposure to the limits of our craft. Interactions between physician and patient are too brief. We need to work toward making our time together more productive. Trust is paramount and may take a while to develop.

The patient needs to arrive with his or her thoughts organized. What questions need to be asked? Is the physician's office the place where answers will be found? Will patients not only list the medications they are taking, but reveal the ones they have long ago abandoned?

Too often, neither the major losses nor the minor frustrations and humiliations of daily life are shared with the physician; this, in part, is due to medically directed questions. Our symptom-oriented review of systems glosses over these important aspects of health and disease.

There is hope for fundamental change. Quality care initiatives include a focus on quality-of-life measurements—patient self-assessment tools that permit physicians to better comprehend the patient's world outside the office setting, as well as their true level of satisfaction with the results of treatment. Electronic communications may provide means for secure, direct, and rapid contact between patient and care provider, allowing for clarification of instructions, quick reporting of adverse reactions, and modification of treatment plans.

We physicians know the less effective our treatments, and the more restricted our knowledge, the more our patients will turn elsewhere for answers. Some individuals with a chronic illness, having little awareness of their medical options, will deny, ignore, or flout their difficulties. Treatments fail because they are not followed, or because side effects are not discussed with regard to possible adjustments or medication changes. Frustration with side effects, expense, or inconvenience, may lead to noncompliance. Hopelessness and depression may result in failure to pursue further treatment or to communicate one's true status honestly and accurately.

Help may be very near at hand. Few individuals encounter problems unique to themselves. Few lack friends, family, and community resources that can allay fears. Disease-specific support groups can become a source of information and emotional support. While attending to a wide range of medical and psychological issues, this author has been able to record the comfort that those close to us can provide.

Can we alter our fate even if we cannot cure our disease? Can we improve the quality of our life? Our ability may be weakened by extreme pain or handicapping conditions. In most instances, however, the individual afflicted with the illness is the one who determines whether he or she is a victim of circumstances or a person with a sense of control over his or her choices. New problems may arise each day. We can surmount these only by calling upon the essential qualities of communication, learning, and love. Bianca Podesta provides a light for the path.

~Lee S. Shapiro, MD, FACP, Director of Scleroderma Clinic at the Center for Rheumatology in Albany and Sarasota, Clinical Associate Professor of Medicine at Albany Medical College, and Winner of National Scleroderma Foundation Distinguished Physician 2007 Lifetime Achievement Award

INTRODUCTION

As is the case with many patients, the diagnosis of scleroderma did not mark the onset of the disease in me. I had some of the symptoms for decades, including esophageal dismotility, Raynaud's Syndrome, sclerodacktyly, and telangiectasias. Of these, Raynaud's and problems with my esophagus were the most serious. With my 2004 diagnosis, questions arose that I was not able to ask aloud: *Will there be changes in my appearance? Will I be dependent on steroids someday? How long do I have to live?*

For the next three years I continued to work part-time in my duel professions as minister and pastoral counselor. Plagued by fatigue and more frightening symptoms, I hid my fears among a growing pile of books. The medical texts were hard to understand; their photographs of patients whose conditions were examples of worse-case scenarios were alarming. Caught between denial and grief, I funneled my feelings into writing a novel.

On May 7, 2008, I sat in a consultation room with my rheumatology specialist, Dr. Lee S. Shapiro. "After the novel is finished" I told him, "I'd like to get started on a book about self-care in scleroderma."

"I can see such a book helping many people," he said. "Why don't you write that one first?"

This brief exchange took place at the end of our appointment time; he was standing near the door, looking down at me. I could see he meant what he said.

I had never written a novel before; while, on the other hand, I had been in the helping business for a long time. If I followed through with this process of daily documentation, study, and reflection, I might not only provide a valuable resource for patients and practitioners, but perhaps draw closer to the possibility of my own healing.

The day after that appointment with my specialist, I began my journal, keying in a detailed account of every symptom I was experiencing with my corresponding, sometimes clumsy, attempts to find relief. Soon, I was writing about work, relationships, and what I was reading and thinking, as well. The journal became a friend that drew me into conversation almost every morning and evening for a year; a year during which I was dealing with a number of scleroderma-related health issues. Excerpts of my journal are used to illustrate the themes in this book. My research included interviews with several people with scleroderma and other autoimmune diseases, review of medical texts and research, and books by other writer/patients.

For more than two years I moved toward an understanding of scleroderma and the effects it has had and may have on my own and on others' lives. My initial goal was to reach out to individuals with scleroderma, encouraging them to respond to medical decisions and self-care practices that may increase the length and quality of their lives. Nurses and physicians among my first readers recognized the information's usefulness to the medical field. Providing an overview of the symptoms of systemic scleroderma and the psychological impact of the disease on patients, who must navigate a labyrinth of choices, gives clinicians and patients a more complete picture of this complex condition.

In the year following my last journal entry in May 2009, I have followed a gluten-free, cow-dairy free diet, and increased my intake of and fondness for green vegetables. I continue to exercise in a group and on my own, according to my physical therapist's recommendations. Fatigue, esophageal issues, Raynaud's Syndrome, and mobility symptoms have improved significantly. This I attribute not only to various lifestyle changes I have been able to make with the help of my friends, co-workers, and medical practitioners, but also to a renewal of my inner life. If I neglect self-care disciplines for even a day, symptoms begin to reappear.

I feel deep gratitude for every person, near and far, who is part of the healing network about which I write and to which I belong.

PART I
PHYSICAL MANIFESTATIONS

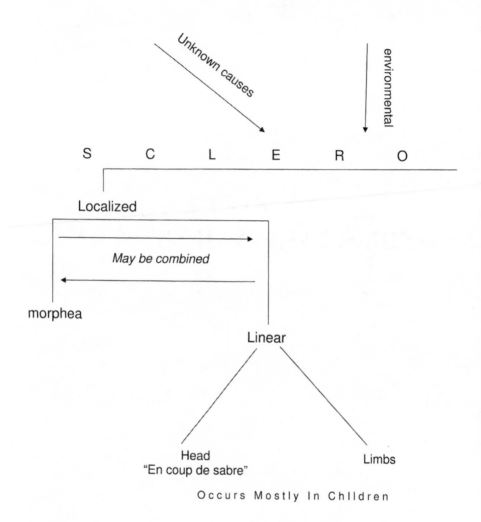

The Scleroderma Map

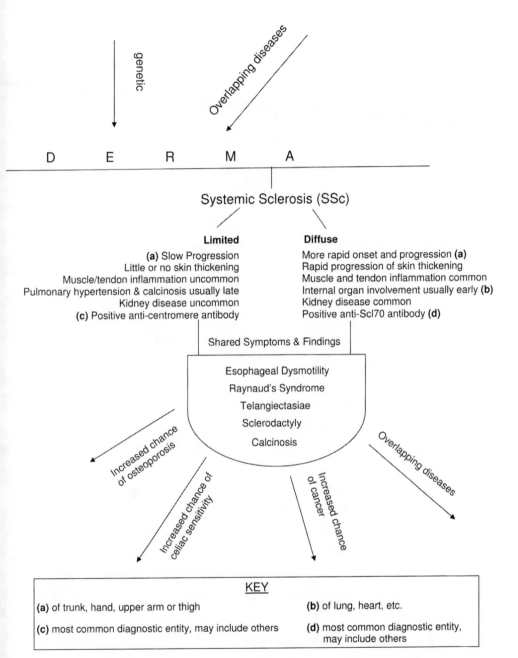

Chapter 1
SKIN

"Your skin is the fingerprint of what's going on in your body…"

~Georgiana Donadio, PhD

For individuals with scleroderma, skin lesions—changes in the skin—reflect problems that are often more than skin deep. Our bodies are made up of multiple interdependent systems, and in every form of scleroderma more than one system is usually involved at the same time.

Skin problems for those with the *limited* form of scleroderma, or systemic sclerosis (SSc), the type with which I have been diagnosed, may be mild to severe:, such as: calcinosis, calcium salt deposits underneath the skin; Raynaud's Syndrome, which presents as multi-colored changes in fingers and toes in reaction to cold or stress; sclerodactyly: hardening of skin on the fingers and toes; esophageal issues; and telengiectasiae, appearing as little red blood vessel spots on hands, feet, or tongue all represent five clues to diagnosis.

Keep in mind that diagnosis in this family of autoimmune connective-tissue diseases is a continuing, often frustrating puzzle because of the possibility of overlapping conditions. The original diagnosis may include, or mutate, into a second autoimmune disease entity in the same person.

The other type of systemic sclerosis, called *diffuse*, can present with painful symptoms that permanently affect the skin and most often involve underlying tissue, muscles, and organs. Swelling and tightness of the hands can sometimes be so extreme as to render them almost useless. Thankfully, with treatment, the swelling usually subsides in a number of months, but the tightness may remain much longer. Itching, called pruritus, may produce levels of pain that are not manageable by application of over-the-counter products. Swelling and tightening of facial skin often evolves to leave wrinkles or crinkly skin around the mouth, and diminished ability to open the mouth.

Even localized scleroderma can bring serious skin issues. *Morphea*, the most common form of localized scleroderma, presents as one or more shiny patches of hard skin, either single or multiple, with different patterns of coloring or pigmentation. Medical intervention varies with regard to the depth, location, and texture of the skin surface involved. These lesions most often soften spontaneously.

The other form of the localized type of scleroderma is called *linear* scleroderma. This occurs most frequently in children and can be disfiguring. If the scar-like "line" extends too deeply underneath the skin, muscle and even bone growth may be affected, resulting in limb-length discrepancy, or facial asymmetry. Although the *linear* type of localized scleroderma rarely includes Raynaud's Syndrome, self-care tips for general skin health that appear in the journal entries may still be helpful.

I found no data about how changes in diet or vitamin supplements can affect skin changes in scleroderma, or about the use of nutritive oils in the restoration of its elasticity and function except in the work of psychic diagnostician, Edgar Cayce.

Cayce, born in 1877, was a renowned healer with no formal education beyond grade school, yet had wide success with thousands of sick people for whom he gave "life readings." While Cayce was in a trance state, lying on a couch at home, with his wife Gertrude opening communications from the patient or the patient's family, his secretary took shorthand notes of his recommendations. Cayce spoke from a deep unconscious state, conveying knowledge that was unknown to his conscious mind.

Two books, *Scleroderma Volume I and II, Circulating Files Extracts from the Edgar Cayce Readings* are about patients diagnosed with scleroderma, some of whom were consulting with physicians as well. These and other publications addressing autoimmune diseases are available from A.R.E., The Association of Research and Enlightenment in Virginia Beach, Virginia.

As a young woman I read a description of applications to the skin involving castor oil as prescribed by Edgar Cayce. This oil has been found in countless instances to restore not only skin cells, but cells beneath the skin.

> Thursday, May 8, 2008
> Swam with the nine a.m. group in the indoor pool of my co-op. Grateful to discover the pre-swim hot shower trick. Pool temperature's maintained at eighty-five degrees; still, Raynaud's attacks in my fingers began in the changing room before I got in the water.

People with scleroderma are often encouraged to swim regularly because swimming does not overstress muscles and joints. Before moving to a building with a pool, finding one close to home was a problem for me. I also had concerns about chlorine and water temperature.

Most heated pools, including the one in my building, have been too cold for my comfort. In Florida's climate, any pool slightly warmer than the current outdoor temperature may be advertised as "heated." Most people with Raynaud's Syndrome have attacks in water cooler than eighty-five degrees. Blue or white fingertips not only ruin the pleasure of swimming, but can harm tissue.

In order to stave off Raynaud's attacks at the pool, I began taking warm-to-hot showers in the changing area immediately before swimming. This made my whole body, core and extremities, warm enough to get into the water without being chilled. The air against my wet skin on the short walk to the pool was easily tolerated because my body core was now warm. This works best if one does not hesitate at the edge, or linger in the lower water, but begins swimming right away.

After a free swim, I take a shower in the changing room, washing with plain glycerin soap and a sponge. Many varieties of store soap may create irritation and itching and sting mucus membranes in the genital/rectal area. When I was a child with no control over my care, I avoided washing because of reacting so painfully to a popular brand of soap my family bought. Although my avoidance of soap and water may have been wiser than I knew, my bathing phobia worried my parents and amused my friends. Since about thirty years ago, when I lost my ability to sweat, a loss common to persons with scleroderma, my avoidance of showering was never a matter of hygiene.

I stay in the sauna just long enough to dry off and smooth on a layer of oil. As long as I can remember, I have applied nutritive oils to my skin after bathing. The oils I use after showering are a mixture of olive and peanut. These oils have a mild scent and are not offensive to others who use the changing area and sauna. Olive oil may make you smell faintly like a salad, while peanut oil is odorless. Castor oil has been ruled unpleasant by some of the women in the swim group who use scented lotions.

Thursday, May 15, 2008

Showed the physician's assistant at my rheumatologist's office the red spots under my tongue, the telangeictsiae, which have been in my mouth for at least twenty years. My former dentist offered to biopsy one of them. Since they had been there as long as I could remember, there seemed no point in having the procedure; though I wonder now if agreeing to the biopsy may have brought me to an earlier diagnosis.

Thursday, May 29, 2008

Checking the outdoor temperatures for the rest of the week, hoping for a warm day at my first Scleroderma Walk. Any reading less than seventy degrees will mean having to wear a hat, gloves, and a turtleneck under my T-shirt.

Saturday, July 5, 2008

Have a new calcinosis site, a little bump under the skin on the inside of my right thumb. Hurts like hell when I take hold of things like exercise weights or my steering wheel. I'm practicing ways of picking up objects to avoid direct contact.

Monday, July 7, 2008

Saw my internist this afternoon. He peered through a lens

at some hard scab-like skin on the edge of my nose and took a swab for analysis. He prescribed a super antibiotic ointment with a back-up of an oral antibiotic in case the ointment does not work within ten days, and/or the area remains painful. A number of doctors and nurses have contracted MRSA, a virulent drug-resistant bacteria, to which I may be vulnerable because of going into hospitals and nursing homes where I touch and am touched by patients. Unlikely the hard flap of skin on my nose is due to scleroderma, he said.

Thursday, July 10, 2008

The sore calcinosis under the skin of my right thumb hasn't bothered me since my hand's learned to pick up and hold things without touching the spot. Now I'm dropping stuff because the new approach interferes with my customary holding response.

Thursday, July 17, 2008

Bob [former husband and current good friend] and I had lunch at the soup place. The AC was frigid. Instead of running to the car for my jacket, I tried creative visualization to adjust my body temperature. Imagined sitting on a hot, sandy beach. By the time the waitress brought the best pea soup in the world, my body felt warmer. Can't rely on biofeedback in every situation, but nice to know the technique works some of the time.

Today helped my housekeeper helper lift a couch on top of the edge of the Oriental rug in the living room. Worked on scouring the extra bathroom; my hands still hurt from the commercial cleaning agents. I need to buy a heavier pair of rubber gloves to protect against Raynaud's.

Saturday, July 26, 2008

Accidentally bumped open the calcinosis on my wrist; awfully sore, draining white calcium salts. Soaked my wrist in warm water with Epsom salts as my local rheumatologist suggested.

Friday, August 8. 2008

Last night at support group, a woman took off her white mitten to show us two fingers ravaged by Raynaud's. I can still picture her one finger, black from first joint to the tip. Another finger was bandaged, appearing dangerously affected, possibly gangrenous. Although the air conditioning in the meeting room didn't seem cold to me, she wore her white mittens the entire hour and a half. She attributed her advanced finger ulcers and other physical setbacks to a year of unusual family stress. I'm going to take Raynaud's attacks and stress more seriously.

Wednesday, September 24, 2008

Sat outside in the warmth of the patio sun for one sweet hour. Back in my apartment, the cooler fall temperatures turned my fingers blue. Trying to put off a Raynaud's attack, held my hands under warm running water. There are permanent changes in my living space I could make to adapt to the colder season. Larger, better quality electric heaters in the kitchen and bedroom would help, even if only for spring and fall.

The necessity for strategies to increase body heat arises because Raynaud's syndrome does not allow for our hands to warm up from circulatory activity. Circulatory activity already has been impaired by small vessel damage. What is required is an external heat source.

Thursday, October 2, 2008

In the car, my furriest gloves couldn't keep my hands

warm, but placing one hand next to my belly skin helped. Also, taking turns putting one hand on the foam-covered steering wheel and the other between my thighs. Although inelegant, this alternation rivals the thickest igloo mittens.

Perhaps the most helpful tip given at the scleroderma support group meeting tonight was the recommendation that, in cold weather, we make use of chemical hand warmers. One member keeps several packets in his car. I've a few stored in a closet which I need to transfer to my glove compartment.

Hand warmers, which are sold in sports and hunting goods stores, come in little packets that fit right into a glove or mitten. Having a glove liner or other protective material between one's skin and the packet is best; I buy a pair of silk glove liners every year for this purpose. When activated, these warmer packets provide steady heat for hours. In the event of a traveling emergency, such as being stuck on a road in winter, they could be finger savers. A construction worker in our group, with the *diffuse* type of scleroderma, uses them regularly. He said storing them in a Ziplock bag directly after wearing permits their re-use a second or third time.

Friday, October 10, 2008

Indian summer. Sat on the patio downstairs, letting the sun shine on my face and arms. Half-blind from the glare, I managed to do paperwork for two hours. What I'll miss most about Florida, if we cannot go this year, is sitting in the sun by the pool. A few years back, the Florida sun stung my skin. Both high temperatures and time of day seem to be factors in whether or not sunlight causes me pain. Today my protection was the cool underpinning of an autumn breeze.

Wednesday, November 19, 2008

Enduring a deep freeze. Came close to a Raynaud's attack before the external heater warmed my counseling office. A friend in my co-op invited me to attend a night class on social justice via the prophets at her synagogue. She offered to drive us from her warm indoor garage space. Touch and go trying to generate body heat in the synagogue's chilly library, but I'm glad I went.

Thursday, November 20, 2008

Almost too cold to go out today. Happily, the pool was nearly bathtub temperature; the sun from the window wall shone on the water. Had to see a few clients and go to the grocery store. My silk glove liners under big ski mittens didn't fend off a Raynaud's attack while picking up fruits and vegetables in the store. Bought a bunch of flowers to lift my spirits.

Sunday, November 23, 2008

Fifty-five degrees in the church where we rehearsed felt like thirty-five. A church staff member said the thermostat read seventy degrees in the choir loft; but we were hundreds of yards away and positioned at a significantly lower level. I wore multiple layers including polyester, cotton, and wool: gloves, tights beneath lined wool trousers, and a hat and scarf. Was still uncomfortably cold most of the three hours except when I put my down coat over everything. Nevertheless, the beautiful music compensated for the drafty chancel. I guess that's why, after twelve winters, I'm still willing to freeze with The Madrigal Choir on occasion. The Choir began more than thirty years ago as a small group dedicated to singing and performing baroque and renaissance music. Although madrigal-style singing remains in our repertoire, we've grown to more than forty members, and perform from a range of musical periods.

Sunday, December 7, 2008

Need to find a way to stay indoors on the coldest days. Dressed in multiple layers, I went out wrapped in a down coat, scarf around face and head, hands in my warmest gloves. After attending the early morning reading group at a local United Methodist church, came home for two hours of leg rest before meeting Bob for Christmas shopping and dinner. Confident in my layering, I walked from store to store in the sub-zero air, wind blowing with Arctic ferocity against eyes and forehead. Secure under all those layers, I had no clue how this would hit me later on. Back home for several awful hours there was a throbbing in my limbs, like a full-body Raynaud's attack.

Some winters ago, I had a more severe reaction. While we practiced processing from the outer church entrance into the sanctuary, we singers in concert dress had to stand in the narthex on a sub-zero, midwinter night. For about fifteen minutes icy air from the street blew through the crack in the huge oak doors, hitting me with scalding intensity, penetrating scarf and hat and cape. To recover from that exposure took most of three days in bed

Monday, December 22, 2008

Drove unfazed more than an hour northwest through the twenty-below-zero windchill. The new thick fold-over flap gloves from the supermarket turned out to be warmer than the expensive ones from the department store. Thankfully, I suffered no hint of Raynaud's.

Sunday, December 28, 2008

Hands much too dry. Right index finger has a crack forming at the tip. Kept castor oil on under stretchy mesh cotton gloves most of the day. So many things waiting to be done, especially the kitchen upgrade before company arrives in a couple of weeks. Keeping hands well oiled and warm a priority.

Wednesday, December 31, 2008

Bob wanted to meet for lunch. Windchill still below zero. I persist in imagining I can overcome the freeze by thoughtful layering. I was exposed to outside air only a few times, going to and from my car, wearing my thickest gloves, and a down-filled fake fur-lined hood worthy of Alaska; after I returned home, recovery took five hours. Hands stayed cold, chest hurt, throat felt as though an icicle had been dropped into it.

Would like to stay in on really cold days. I'd like to have a cut-off point, when the temperature's under fifteen degrees Fahrenheit, for instance. Wish I could tell friends, clients, co-workers I have to cancel on those days because of the weather.

Thursday, January 15, 2009

One of the coldest days of the year. Had to go out twice, once to see clients and pick up a few things at the store. Bundled from head to toe, I wore sandals with compression tights and wool socks. My new manly orthotic-friendly shoes do not fit right in the heel. Glad there's no Raynaud's in my toes.

Being especially careful about getting enough protein, layering, and completely covering face and hands. The windchill provoked Raynaud's attack just the same.

Saturday, January 31, 2009

Colder than expected, frequent Raynaud's attacks over a period of three hours. Wore my warmest gloves, but should have worn silk liners with the chemical warmer inserts. Finding it hard to organize use of the chemical warmers. There is so much time-consuming detail to protect myself from the weather in winter; my good intentions often fail.

Wednesday, February 11, 2009

A perfectly lovely freak of a spring day lifted the spirits of everyone I met. Both the sore spot at the tip of my index finger and the crack in my thumb have healed.

Friday, April 17, 2009

Friend Lynn and I talked about skin sensitivities today.

Lynn, a nurse practitioner, worked full time in a busy medical practice after the onset of multiple sclerosis. Today, we were wondering aloud whether or not skin sensitivities might accompany most autoimmune diseases. Lynn happens to have contact dermatitis and is careful selecting cleaning agents. She applies only baby oil or petroleum jelly to her skin. Other products have caused itching and dry patches. She has never used olive or castor oils, my long-time standbys, and cannot tolerate face makeup.

Wednesday, April 29, 2009

Arriving at the monastery yesterday for time out, I was thrilled by midsummer temperatures. Today's much cooler. Brought in my small electric hand heater from the car. Will need a more powerful heat source if the chill persists.

Monday, May 4, 2009

Today's discovery: By applying oil an hour before my pre-swim shower, I'm protected from the chlorine while swimming. In the shower afterwards, still some residue on arms and legs. That's okay. Peanut oil is the charm.

SELF-CARE OPTIONS

Food

A variety of good foods nourishes skin. Little or no refined sugar and no empty carbohydrates are optimal for skin and all body organs. Healthful fats and oils found in avocado and wild ocean fish nourish skin and rebuild cells.

A balance of food-based B complex, vitamins E, and C may be helpful. Trying to get most or all these nutrients from whole foods and vegetable juices is better than taking an array of supplements. As interest and finances permit, consider vitamins and/or supplements prescribed or recommended by your physician, chiropractor, or nutritionist. Listen closely to your body in determining the effect any new product.

Exercise

Regular exercise is likely to improve circulation in hands and feet and may reduce the number and severity of Raynaud's attacks.

Weight-bearing exercise may broaden venous pathways narrowed as a result of scleroderma. A slight varicosity developing in my right forearm became an ideal location for insertion of the IV during two medical procedures, without pain or bruising.

Upper-body work, such as lifting appropriate weights in the overhead press as well as downward arm motions, stimulates blood flow to hands and fingers. Specific exercises that include intentional stretching can loosen tightened skin around affected areas.

Sleep

A regular sleep pattern of seven-to-eight hours a night promotes restoration of all cells, including those of our skin. According to yogi lore, the most restorative sleep is between ten p.m. and two a.m.

Calcinosis

Soaking the affected area in warm water with Epsom salts may offer relief as long as the skin is unbroken. Draining from calcinosis most often occurs when deposits that have formed over pressure points on the hands, elbows, or knees are rubbed or bumped against a hard surface. For more severe cases, surgical intervention may be advised. Once the sites are healed over, applying nutritive oils or a prescribed cream before bed may promote healing.

More work is involved when applying castor oil packs to calcinosis sites. If applications are carried out according to Cayce's method, with your doctor's approval, this may be the most effective of remedies. (*See* Glossary for instructions for applying castor oil pack.)

Application of antibiotic or other prescribed ointments may be used. I have followed each of the above recommendations when treating a calcinosis site that has drained several times over the past five years. At present, the site is reduced to a single, pale protrusion.

Raynaud's Syndrome

Layered clothing in both warm and colder temperatures is standard for people with primary Raynaud's Syndrome or systemic scleroderma. Carry mittens with liners as well as chemical warmers, especially during the colder seasons. When going outside on the coldest days, cover all parts of face and body except the eyes with a knitted mask or hood and soft scarf.

One hundred percent cotton is the fabric kindest to skin and mucus membranes. Inflammation and itching can arise from wearing underclothing made from a cotton polyester mix or other synthetic materials.

While dishwashing and house-cleaning, nutritive oils or prescribed creams worn under rubber gloves provide therapeutic protection for hands.

Sometimes Raynaud's symptoms and other reactivity to cold and dampness may increase due to under-activity of the thyroid gland. Consult with a physician about the appropriateness of a blood test to check thyroid function.

Pruritus or Itching

Avoid scratching; apply calamine or prescribed lotions after a shower at night or when itching is intense. Do not use harsh soaps and detergents. A mild glycerin-based soap for bath and showering is best. Taking the opportunity for a warm bath in soap-less, non-chlorinated well or spring water followed by a rubdown with a nutritive oil, such as olive or peanut, may be extremely beneficial.

Whenever possible, use natural cleaning supplies for your home: baking soda, white vinegar, mild detergent, lemon extract; or enzyme-based liquid cleaners.

Sun Exposure

Know your skin type and tolerance. If there is a sense of burning pain, stay out of the sun except in moderate weather. Inquire about vitamin-B-complex supplementation, which may strengthen the skin's ability to tolerate sunlight.

Hydration

Drink plenty of filtered, well, or spring water. Drinking alcohol dehydrates the skin; avoid or eliminate.

Do not submerge skin in chlorinated water, or shower more than a few times a week. Rubbing natural oil on the skin before a pre-swim shower and swimming may help protect the skin. Choose pleasant-smelling nutrient lubricants and oils where others are sharing the pool area. Walnut and peanut oils are odorless; a mild cologne may be added to them. Olive oil does not have a strong odor, but does have a food smell. Castor oil, derived from a bean, has a slightly medicinal scent; and its odor is hard to remove from sweat suits and fabrics worn next to the skin. These fabrics may require a soap and baking soda wash.

Since many people with scleroderma do not sweat in areas of thickened skin, showering two to three times a week is usually enough.

The same rules apply to hair and scalp care. Alternate several natural shampoo products once or twice a week. Stay away from all products that are not water soluble; avoid or eliminate sprays, electric hair dryers, and permanent waves.

Don't smoke. Smoking can interfere with blood vessel function and breathing, both of which affect the general health and appearance of the skin.

Cosmetics

Stay with water-soluble, allergen-free make-up products.

Lipstick: If you have celiac disease or gluten sensitivity and follow a gluten-free diet, check the ingredients for trace wheat or other flour products. Some of the cheaper brands contain castor oil, which is all right. More expensive brands, especially those that are advertised as long-lasting, may be more likely to contain harsh chemicals and cause irritation. Once a week wipe the surface of lipsticks with rubbing alcohol. Cosmetics can accumulate harmful bacteria.

Good concealing agents for the skin are easy to obtain. The little red spots from the dilation of small blood vessels near the skin's surface, telangiectasiae, can be covered with hypo-allergenic spot sticks and creams.

Chapter 2
MUSCULOSKELETAL

"The breaking wave and the muscle as it contracts obey the same law. Delicate line gathers the body's total strength in a bold balance. Shall my soul meet so severe a curve, journeying on its way to form?"

~Dag Hammarskjold

Bones, Muscles, Tendons, Nerves

Scleroderma can put stress on the body's infrastructure, the basis of which is our skeletal frame. Although not a primary target of this disease, bones may suffer deep scarring from the *linear* type of localized scleroderma. In more serious cases of *morphea*, which presents as pigmented patches of skin, the underlying soft tissue and muscle can be affected. Extensive contractures, the permanent bending inward of fingers, toes, elbow, or knee joints, sometimes accompany the later stages of the systemic forms. When this occurs, hands may become unable to grasp, or limbs to bend, creating severe handicapping conditions.

Women in midlife make up the largest population of those diagnosed with scleroderma. This is the time leading into menopause; so naturally, there are concerns about bone density. Weight loss, which also may involve loss of bone density, may be difficult to avoid in persons with systemic scleroderma. Taking calcium citrate and vitamin D, as well engaging in a program of regular weight-bearing exercise, are believed to help maintain, and possibly increase density, even after bone thinning or osteopenia has begun.

Myopathy is the medical term for any adverse effects in muscle.

Scleroderma can cause mild-to-moderate muscle pain and stiffness. In the case of less common overlapping syndromes, or in the setting of unintentional weight loss, severe muscle wasting may occur. This may lead to interruptions in basic functioning; since our muscles not only hold the skeletal frame in place, but enable us to wash, feed, and dress ourselves. However, the most common occurrence in long-term patients is a mild atrophy, which regular exercise may keep from worsening.

Striated muscles are muscles that move by conscious control. Regulated by the higher nervous system, they respond to our will under normal circumstances. Before we move, for instance, we decide to lift a glass of water or to climb the stairs.

Smooth muscle, on the other hand, operates independently of conscious control or intention; and is involved in the working of our heart muscle, breathing mechanism(s), and the movements that propel our food downward along the entire path of the digestive tract. In those with the systemic forms of scleroderma, loss of smooth muscle elasticity and function may have an adverse affect on the circulatory, pulmonary, and/or digestive systems.

Joints and tendons also figure into the progressive nature of the systemic forms of this disease. Inflammation may cause pain similar to that caused by true arthritis; as well as stiffness in wrists, elbows, or knees. Contractures are common. At the mildest, fingers as well as arms and legs may not extend to their full length or flex as fully as they should. At the extreme, limbs may be forced into distortions that prohibit normal function. The swelling of fingers and toes and the tightness of skin and tendons also may limit joint motion.

Tendons secure the muscles to our bones. While persons with scleroderma may show symptoms of tendonitis and bursitis, which are common in the general population, people with systemic sclerosis can develop something called tendon rub. *Tendon rubs* are the consequence of a stiffening or thickening of the fibrous sheath that surrounds the tendon and normally helps to buffer the joints from movement and the impacts of daily life. People with tendon thickening often can hear or feel a dull rubbing when bending their wrists, fingers, ankles, and shoulders. Less commonly, the tendon sheath will calcify or rupture.

Nerves send signals of pain, pleasure, numbness, or tingling from points of tension, inflammation, or other trauma. There are four major nerve issues, or *neuropathies*, in scleroderma. *Cranial neuropathies* refer to places in the face or head served by this major cranial pathway. The most common is *Bell's palsy* where pressure from arthritic or inflammatory narrowing causes a loss of sensation on the affected side and the ability to move muscles that surround the eye and mouth. Bell's palsy has been known to reverse spontaneously, but may leave a discernable trace.

Another nerve category is *entrapment neuropathies*. These occur often near a joint where, due to fibrosis or hardening, a neural pathway has been narrowed, resulting in pain and possible dysfunction. *Carpal tunnel syndrome* is the best known entrapment neuropathy, in which case the wrist and hand become painful and/or difficult to move.

Peripheral or *sensorimotor neuropathies* are different from the others. These cause numbness and tingling and may be the consequence of fibrosis and narrowing or inflammation in a blood vessel supplying the nerve. Left unchecked, in extreme cases, occlusion, or blockage, of a blood vessel can cause death of a nerve, resulting in the inability for it to supply sensation or to prompt muscle action. *Foot drop*, where the ankles cannot be lifted up in walking is a particular hazard of this type of nerve damage.

The fourth category is damage to *autonomic nerves*, nerves which control bladder and bowel function (discussed in Chapter 3).

As with all bodily systems, the first line of musculoskeletal self-care is a balance of good nutrition, sleep, and exercise. Alternative approaches to healing include various remedies from application of oils to nutritional supplements, some of which will be discussed in the following narrative and journal notes. In the event that mobility is threatened or impaired, physical therapy, surgery, and/or steroids may be recommended and/or prescribed.

Wednesday, May 14, 2008

Osteoporosis showed up in three places on my bone-density test, my right arm, left hip, and lower spine. Since esophageal problems preclude my taking prescribed oral medication for bone density, my scleroderma specialist recommended an intravenous drug, which I could receive every few months at my local rheumatologist's office.

Thursday, May 15, 2008

Been thinking about the Scleroderma Walk, imagining how much easier riding would be than walking. Began to search for a bike and was attracted to the lean lines of a blue tricycle on the main floor of the bicycle shop. Sat for a while on the seat, thinking how I could attach a flag or sign, acknowledging the generosity of the shop's owner, a guy named Joe who agreed to try to lend me one for this year's Scleroderma Walk.

Friday, May 16, 2008

Last night I had a dream in which I was climbing stairs. My leg muscles were hurting; I was having trouble getting up each step. When I awoke, I began again to think about the IV treatment for bone density with reported side effects of muscle aches. My muscles already ache!

A problem churning in my mind for a while seems to attract answers out of the blue, like an electrical current miraculously finding its likeness in a sea of multiple currents. For instance, when I was working out this afternoon, a neighbor showed up in the exercise room. Ten years my junior, she's already suffered a severe hip fracture from osteoporosis. When I asked about her treatment, she mentioned taking the IV therapy I've been thinking about. Like me, she's been taking a proton-pump inhibitor (PPI), a common acid-inhibiting drug, for a number of years. We'd both read how long-term use of these drugs may inhibit the absorption of calcium.

Another instance: A few days ago, I asked a friend who's an RN about the IV drug on my mind. She mailed me a newspaper article reporting incidences of necrosis of the jaw, particularly in women who have had numerous root canals and other serious dental issues, as well as among some women with autoimmune diseases. Necrosis means death—death of the jaw. I've come a long way from dreaming about muscle aches. An arduous history of dental and gum problems may put me at the back of the line for the recommended IV therapy. A single contraindication for this drug would not be so bad, but having long-term dental problems as well as a serious autoimmune disease, a disease which may have contributed to those dental issues, is a double whammy. I know I'm imagining the worst-case scenario; but if I had a choice between the inability to walk and the inability to chew, speak, and smile, I would begin shopping for a wheelchair right away.

Saturday, May 17, 2008

Restorative hours at home to putter and rest. Enjoyed this morning's phone conversation with my son. After hearing about my osteoporosis, he asked whether I believe that dairy products deliver absorbable calcium. He's not convinced and I'm not sure myself. His family by marriage is Japanese American. A glance into their refrigerator reveals minimal consumption of milk and cheese compared to most American families. Although not strict vegetarians, their daily staples are fresh vegetables, eggs, and grains, with rice and soy products predominating. On special occasions, wild baked or grilled salmon. Sushi restaurants are birthday celebration destinations.

Sunday, May 18, 2008

Max and Geri drove some distance to hear The Madrigal Choir's concert of Welsh sacred music. Dinner at my apartment afterwards, laughing and telling stories. The aftermath was not so wonderful. Too much time on my feet: first, during the singing, then the cooking. They left around 7:30. After half an hour of cleaning up, I'd become quite crippled. Ordinarily

I'm asleep by 10:30, but pain in my hips, accompanied by foot cramps, kept me awake. At midnight, I went to the kitchen, took a mild sleeping aid and was out in half an hour.

Monday, May 19, 2008

Woke at 6:00 feeling much better, leg and hip pain gone. Just the same, scolding myself for overdoing. Aim to be more careful, to have a smoother week with better pacing.

Sunday, May 25, 2008

Need to be more intentional about weight-bearing exercise. Swimming's not enough. Working out on the stationary bike and rowing machine feels good, but am I building bone? My chiropractor told me to find a tested system. Wish there were a way to make weight-lifting more interesting. How can I fit the practice into my schedule?

Friday, June 6, 2008

Today's my son's birthday. Wish they didn't live so far away. After a slow beginning, I rode the stationary bike. If I didn't have so much muscle pain, I could put the apartment in order. My legs hurt from walking around the stores after only a small amount of shopping for cards and food items. Afterwards, I lay on the bed for most of the evening, not wanting to stand or walk. I'd like to do some straightening up before working on Sunday's message. Being a pastor with a limp is okay; they don't expect ballet.

Wednesday, July 4, 2008

Vitamin-D blood level, which had been low, is closer to normal after only six weeks of taking the D supplement and calcium capsules from my chiropractor. He told me again if I am disciplined about weight-bearing exercise, I might see a significant increase in bone density in about six months. He keeps telling me the same thing; I guess I'm the one who's avoiding. At this point, I'm not a walker; it hurts too much. After an hour on my feet, I need to rest. Weight-lifting? Barbells?

Thursday, December 4, 2008

I was already beginning to fade before the scleroderma support group's holiday party began. After a couple of hours, my right leg and knee were so painful I had to lean on chairs while walking from place to place. In spite of my temporary crippling, the spirit of the evening brought great pleasure.

Tuesday, December 9, 2008

According to my Albany rheumatologist, my knee pain's probably not scleroderma related. He suggested a consult with an orthopedist. Keep thinking the knee pain may have something to do with ligaments because of my maternal great grandmother. Only a suspicion, but I recall her complaining about "torn ligaments." Sometimes she used a cane or leaned on the surrounding furniture when she walked around, the way I've been doing. When the maternal side of my family lived together in a three-story townhouse, I remember her lying on her bed for hours every afternoon to rest her legs.

Coincidentally, I found out this afternoon that ligaments appear to be the reason. My chiropractor said surgical repair for a tear can take up to a year in a hard brace to heal. He wrapped my knee with a canvas ice-pack, which stayed on for ten minutes, and applied ultrasound therapy. He sent for an elastic brace for when I'm planning to be on my feet more than an hour. He said after the pain is gone, muscle strengthening would help. Here I am again with a recommendation to build muscle strength and no clear directive. My responsibility, I guess, to research possibilities. My interest is strong, but my energy's at an all-time low.

Wednesday, December 10, 2008

Nathalie called—my longest enduring friend. Brief conversation before we had to go. She has a knee problem, too. Her knee may require replacement; though, for the time being, exercise and homeopathy's working fine.

Saw the shoe-fitting specialist who, in considering my spinal curvature, believes proper orthotic and shoe depth may help take pressure off the knee. I've been through this before. My bedroom closet contains an archive of orthotic shoe inserts.

I'm following my chiropractor's suggestion to do three ten-minute applications of ice on the swollen area below my knee. A large bag of frozen peas molds nicely around any limb. He suggested I support the knee with ACE bandages over compression hose, which I'm also doing. Still hurts.

The exercise room's off-limits until I have the brace. Attempted to use my desk chair as a temporary wheelchair to do household chores without putting weight on my knee. No solution. Swam for half an hour.

Sunday, December 14, 2008

No therapeutic nap, no frozen peas on my knee, no nice vegetable with lamb shank supper distracted me from my ruminations. While I cleaned, while I wrapped presents, even while I was making some routine phone calls, couldn't stop thinking about how a pain in the knee or anywhere else in the body is never simply what it seems. This knee pain could be related to previous injuries and influencing my body's limbs and balance. A new pain brings to consciousness old pains, in much the same way that a new grief brings up old grief.

So, I run down the list: On the foot of the right leg with the bum knee, there's a sore toe from an inflamed corn; a large bunion sits on the big toe; above, a weakened ankle from a bad sprain twenty years ago. The central interference with mobility, however, is my spine that is curved like a long S on the X-ray, though I exercise every day in order to stand and sit straighter. Last, but not least, I fell on the right side of head and hip while playing touch football a couple of months ago in L.A. Another souvenir from the same trip is a lingering ache along my right shoulder.

Wondering if awareness of the old injuries to the right side of my body may be a clue about how to treat the weakest link where it hurts the most—in this case, my right knee. At least, this review teases me into thinking I may have some control over the matter.

Tuesday, December 16, 2008

Last night read "Super Healing" by Julie L. Silver, M.D., an essay, adapted from her book by the same title (Rodale Press, 2007), that was printed in the Nov/Dec 2008 issue of *The Magazine A.A.R.P.* She writes about how our bodies have the ability to repair themselves after various types of trauma or injury, and outlines ways we can tap into this power. Her three recommendations are: nutritious foods, enough sleep, and appropriate exercise. All three are basic to self-care; yet, as we all know, any one of these may seem impossible to obtain.

Silver advises that we attempt to obtain most of the vitamins we need for healing from the foods we eat. She's a proponent of the once-a-day multivitamin in which I have never had much faith; although I've heard that taking a multivitamin before or after a large meal may help with digestion. She does allow for some people who have special needs to take extra vitamins or minerals, particularly calcium.

Silver's suggestion most timely for me is *Bromelain*, made from a mixture of enzymes found in fresh pineapple, an isolate which is known to reduce bruising, swelling, and pain. In my thirties and forties, I ate fresh pineapple to treat my frequent respiratory ailments as well as back pain. I'm wondering if my knee might benefit from some fresh pineapple. There's little perceptible swelling, but plenty of pain.

Sunday, December 21, 2008

Faithful with the pineapple, the hot, wet terrycloth against my knee under the frozen peas, and the warm castor oil packs. Castor oils' indelible stains are on everything from my old bathing suits to bedsheets. The knee's better if I put compression hose on first thing in the morning. For two days I've not needed the ACE bandage.

Part of my knee problem may be the sizing of my right orthotic insert. The shoe-fitting expert said the right heal base as too high, which causes the right foot to be propelled forward. Tomorrow I will talk it over with my chiropractor. He should know more about the interdependence of the body's balance mechanisms than the shoe man. Logical to suspect damaged knee ligaments will not have much chance to heal if I'm creating extra stress by walking on an uneven base.

Thursday, January 1, 2009

A full day working at home, a late workout with no nap, tired bones looking toward bed. I can prepare for Sunday's service while reclining, feet and legs elevated and warm.

Just read an article in the July 2008 *Mayo Clinic Health Letter*, (Volume 27, #7), that addresses edema, specifically swelling in the legs. Although the fluid around my knee is slight, I want to do everything I can to make it go away. One of the directives is sodium restriction; my blood tests have always shown a fairly high level of sodium. Still doing the exercises, the peas, compression stockings—the works. Now, life without salt?

Friday, February 6, 2009

I'd like to be able to stay inside during the coldest weather or else live in a warmer climate through the worst of winter.

Saturday, February 21, 2009

I lay on the massage table not for eliminating a specific pain, although before today's treatment still had the ache in my left shoulder from last fall's touch football injury. Mostly curious to understand how this form of hands-on treatment might promote healing in any body suffering from chronic pain, as in scleroderma.

Sunday, February 22, 2009

Benefits from yesterday's body massage continue. For the first time since my twenties I'm enjoying the complete absence of pain. Throughout my adult life I've learned to ignore various levels of discomfort. After a look at my spine, an orthopedic doctor once told me I'd be on pain medication the rest of my life. A terrifying prediction, and I'm glad he was wrong. My coping strategies at that time were greatly in need of improvement. As a young woman I drank to blur the edges. When liquor made me sick, I went to a counselor. Psychotherapy couldn't take away the pain, but did help me to relax and, eventually, to respect the importance of self-care. Of course, there were emotional issues also drawing me to therapy: first, as a patient, then, as a graduate student in psychology. For starters, there was the wonderment about why I took so long to grow up. Much of my life I felt like a five-year-old masquerading as an adult. Treatment went on for seven years before I settled into some ease with who I am.

In my late thirties, a series of losses led to my spiritual renewal, to theological study, and to my work as a congregational minister. Intermittent joint and muscle pain was always there, yet never stopped me from learning or serving. At seminary, I got permission to lie on a foam mat during lectures because I could not sit for more than a half hour in the student desks. Disciplines that helped to soothe my own and others' pain helped me to embrace the good around and within me. I learned to work through minor discomforts, whether located in shoulder, back, leg, foot, or mind. Now I can sit in a chair for longer than an hour, although I shouldn't. If I don't get up every half hour and move around, the stiffness and achy joints come on and I move like an actor playing the part of a very old person.

Tuesday, March 24, 2009

At my invitation, Lynn, my friend with M.S., and I met in a little restaurant which went from quiet and private to loud and public fifteen minutes after our arrival. We compared notes on how our diseases, categorized as autoimmune, could be related and how we might learn from each other.

Friday, April 17, 2009

After a little nap, went to visit Lynn. We sat on her deck for two hours. Our conversation covered the gamut on a day so warm I took off my turtleneck and wore just my tank top. We were having such a good time sitting in the sun, keeping focused on the reason for our meeting wasn't easy. How we are each trying to stay as well while living with a chronic disease.

Lynn stresses the importance of exercise. Every morning she walks from seven-thirty to eight-thirty, rain or shine, snow or sleet. She takes a class once a week in yoga to which she attributes her flexibility and nerve balance. Osteoarthritis and rheumatoid arthritis, generic traits, keep her purposefully exercising her hands and fingers, exercises she was taught by a physical therapist.

Lynn is the rare individual who can claim that all her life she enjoyed a wholesome diet. Her mother, a nurse, took nutrition seriously and consistently provided a variety of healthful foods, as Lynn does now for her family. She takes no vitamins or supplements except a calcium and vitamin D every night to maintain bone health.

The onset of Lynn's multiple sclerosis came while she was working full time at a clinic. Nerves, muscles and joints, GI tract, respiratory system, vision, and organ involvement all can be affected by MS. For about a week Lynn lost all feeling in her trunk and lower body. She continued to work during this week-long crisis. Why?

"What is most important to us is who we are," she said. She was referring to not abandoning the work to which she was dedicated and identified, even for a week.

The clinic staff supported her. They were colleagues in the truest sense, offering help in whatever way they could, while she came in every day, not knowing how or when her situation would be resolved. For nights, she hired a nurse to care for her at home.

Lynn believes her hourly walk each morning is what keeps her moving. If she neglects walking for even a day, she is afraid she may not be able get up out of a chair. She continues walking in the dead of winter, not excluding sub-zero days. Cold does not bother her, she said; she can bundle up and stay warm enough.

Monday, April 27, 2009

Erect posture supports musculoskeletal health. Not sure what to do to improve mine. A few wall push-ups, leg lifts, and yoga poses on the floor every day, nothing intense. In recent months I've been too weak to take on more ambitious exercise.

Thursday, May 1, 2009

Here I am at the monastery on the mountaintop; my week to rest, to meditate, to invite the Spirit. An aching knee and protracted recovery from an esophageal ulcer pushed my bone density issue into the background until this afternoon when the guillotine fell. The doctor's cell phone message about this year's bone scan put me to bed. I've reached an impasse. The calcium and vitamin D, the exercises, did not do what I'd hoped they would. After a year of making skeletal strength a priority, I've failed the test—and kept a careful record of how not to build new bone.

Am I the only one who regresses to a child state when disappointed? I lay down on my bed under quilt and crucifix and wept softly into my pillow. My heart cried out to all those saints who are believed to inhabit this windy, holy place.

Friday, May 15, 2009

Today, I went for the first time to a twice-weekly class designed to increase or maintain existing bone density. Several women from my building attend the group whose members range in age from their sixties upward. A trained leader teaches the exercises and checks our form. With my doctor's note of approval, I'll be able to lift hand weights as well as strapping a weight to my ankle for the leg lifts.

Members of the class have developed a bond, maybe because of our shared objective. We count together to accompany each exercise. Our voices in unison sound almost like a chant. One woman, who closes her eyes for the counting, says the practice brings her into a meditative state. During break time, we have a drink of water and visit. There have been certified successes of increased bone density among the participants. I hope this will happen for me.

SELF-CARE OPTIONS

Compression Hosiery

I had been wearing moderate compression hose for twenty years before my SSc diagnosis. They were prescribed to keep my varicosities from becoming larger and more painful. Since experiencing significant pain in my knee and hip, wearing support hose from morning until night has provided the additional benefit of enabling me to be on my feet for a longer time. I take them off when I lie down to rest or nap during the day.

Warning: Because compression hosiery, if too tight or improperly fitted, can cause blood clots or other vascular problems, consult first with your physician and have experienced medical supply personnel measure you for correct fit.

Nutrition

Consider inquiring of your physician about changing to a gluten-free diet. Whether or not one tests positive in a blood test for celiac sensitivity, omission of wheat flour and gluten is believed to halt or to reverse osteoporosis in many women. In Dr. John O. A. Pagano's book *One Cause, Many Ailments, Leaky Gut Syndrome* (A.R.E. Press, 2008), he cites the linkage between celiac or gluten sensitivity and osteoporosis. Malabsorption issues are evident in gluten-sensitive individuals. Vitamin D and calcium, both of which are needed for bone growth, may be among the nutrients their bodies are unable to absorb. In fact, practitioners that promote natural healing are beginning to regard osteoporosis itself as an immune disease entity. A gluten-free diet is recommended by naturopathic doctors as well for persons with autoimmune diseases.

Vitamins D and calcium are essential to bone health. The easiest form of calcium to absorb and to take is calcium citrate, the gold standard of calcium supplements. The powder form, available in health food stores, is more economical than tablets or capsules and can be mixed with applesauce or yogurt. Dividing up the daily dosage is wise, as the body can utilize only 350 to 400 units at a time. For persons who may be lactose intolerant, milk products can be replaced by servings of goat feta cheese, buttermilk, and yogurt, all believed to boost calcium absorption if eaten around the time calcium supplement is taken.

To determine whether or not you are getting enough calcium and vitamin D, request testing for these along with any regular blood-work order. While sunlight is a natural converter of vitamin D when absorbed by the skin, for persons with scleroderma who experience pain from the sun, the sunlight source is contraindicated.

Nutritive Oils

Several times a week I rub my arms and legs with peanut oil, focusing on tender or sore muscles. When needed, I apply castor oil packs with a hot water bottle over stiff or painful joints. To test whether allergies or reactions to a particular oil, apply a small amount to the inside of your forearm a day or two before beginning regular use or applying a pack.

Physical Therapy

Physical therapy can reverse muscular atrophy or insufficiency. Unlike exercise classes, martial arts, and other elective body work, physical therapy is tailored to one's particular medical needs. A rheumatologist or primary physician can evaluate and refer. Such a referral has been very helpful to me for increasing strength and flexibility, and reversing atrophy in my left leg.

Doctors become accustomed to people who prefer easy solutions. They may not be forthcoming with a recommendation or referral to physical therapy because this time-consuming process may result in only temporary relief. Positive outcomes from physical therapy may last less than a week after the prescribed exercises are stopped. Continuation of these exercises at home is the patient's responsibility.

Stretching

Yoga and Tai Chi are two excellent disciplines for persons with scleroderma. Qigong, a slow discipline widely practiced in China, has stirred recent interest in the U.S. Joining a group to exercise is usually easier than trying to learn on one's own. Modifications may be necessary for those who have difficulties with balance or the ability to extend one's limbs fully.

While serving churches in New Jersey, I had a horizontal pole installed in a doorway of my home for hanging and swinging from my arms and doing chin-ups. My goal was to straighten my slightly bowed spine.

Strontium

The introduction of strontium citrate into my diet was inspired by the poor results in my spring 2009 bone density test. This supplement, used for bone health, has been a popular medicinal in Europe since the early 1800s. Not to be confused with the contaminating Strontium 90 from radioactive fallout in the 1950s this natural element is chemically similar to calcium. There have been studies in both Sweden and the U.S., proving efficiency in promoting bone density in post menopausal women.

Nevertheless, caution informs my method. My naturopathic doctor suggested I begin taking three capsules a day, at least an hour separate from any of my three calcium dosages or other mineral-containing supplements. Because strontium has a slight chance of causing unwelcome side effects in the kidneys, which are vulnerable organs in a percentage of persons with scleroderma, I take only one capsule of 227 mgs.

Swimming

This exercise is easy on joints and an enjoyable way of moving in a field of lighter gravity.

Weight-bearing exercise

In every small city there are several groups that teach and supervise bone-building exercises. Some of these classes may be found in residential health facilities as osteoporosis is prevalent in the aging population. This provides a less expensive alternative to hiring a personal trainer from a health club, and a good way, if one is able, to maintain strength and mobility.

Chapter 3
DIGESTION

"Edible substances evoke the secretion of thick, concentrated saliva. Why?
The answer, obviously, is that this enables the mass of food to pass smoothly
through the tube leading from the mouth into the stomach."

~ Ivan Pavlov

MOUTH, DENTAL, AND THROAT

The alimentary tract represents a long journey from the entrance at the
mouth to the exit at the anus. In people with a systemic form of scleroderma,
limited or *diffuse*, there is an eighty-to-ninety percent chance of digestive
difficulties along the way. This is lamentable not only because of the
inconvenience and pain of gastrointestinal problems. Since infancy, we have
developed a strong emotional connection between food and love. Eating is
much more than salivating and taking in fuel for our bodies. At best, eating is
a source of pleasure, of social sharing, a renewal of one's being. Eating can be
a stress buster or a source of stress, depending upon how well we are able to
deal with temporarily handicapping gastrointestinal events, which may occur
over the course of our illness.

Chewing is the first step in the digestive process. Thorough chewing,
while strongly encouraged, can be difficult when mouth or dental problems
are present. Dry mouth is common in scleroderma and may be present with
or without a diagnosis of *Sjogren's Syndrome*. *Sjogren's*, a disease that often
overlaps with scleroderma, involves the drying of mucus membranes. One
who is unaffected can hardly imagine how having to sip water or another

liquid to moisten every bite of food must interfere with the pleasure of eating.

Many prescribed and over-the-counter medications list dry mouth as a common side effect. Without the protective presence of saliva, teeth readily become targets for decay and/or loosening. Visits to the dentist's office for checkups and supervision of oral hygiene may become more frequent, as these exams, combined with at-home dental care are the best defense against tooth loss.

There are other causes of dental vulnerability in scleroderma. Persons with decreased oral aperture, or narrowed mouth, have trouble opening wide enough for the dentist to carry out repair and other corrective procedures. Cellular changes evidenced by the hardening of gum tissue can interfere with the injection of local anesthesia. Density of gum tissue may interfere also with the numbing of the cranial nerves central to blocking pain.

Long-time usage of prescription narcotics for pain management, as well as stomach acid splashing up through the esophagus and into the throat and mouth from GERD, may result in tooth loss that no amount of brushing and flossing is able to prevent.

Maintaining our teeth, whether they are the originals, implants, or well-fitting dentures, is the first step toward good digestion.

Monday, May 12, 2008

8:15 a.m. in the dentist's chair, having just been given the first injection of the local anesthetic for a root canal. Even though my dentist applied an analgesic before inserting the needle, the pain was pretty intense. The dentist's attempt to numb via the quadrant, a sort of neural hub, didn't work. I have a lot of scar tissue in my gums from years of dental repairs and procedures. After a few more tries, he began drilling, while talking me through the ordeal.

"You're going to be fine," he said. "And a little more of the anesthetic…"

Countless injections, but the nerve in question remains lively. My lip, which used to be the proof of drilling readiness, can still feel the press of his finger. He's added shots all around the affected tooth: four or five, eight or ten, I lost count.

Giving up on the anesthesia, I stiffened my torso against moving while he worked. Every time he got near the nerve, I tightened every muscle in neck and back in order to remain motionless. Tears began to fall sideways down my cheeks.

He stopped. When I was thirty and lived in New York City, I was given nitrous oxide gas, which transported me to another planet—and this at a time when the local anesthetic was still effective. At last he announced he would have to shoot the painkiller directly into to the pulp of the nerve in order to complete cleaning of the canal. With his apologies in the background, I experienced a momentary excruciation worse than I can remember from all my years in dentist chairs.

When he saw that the final needle was effective, there was much scraping and drilling. His assistant kept busy with the suction. Totally relaxed, no longer anticipating pain, I almost fell asleep. On the edge of consciousness, I thought about people with pain that never goes away, who can never fully rest or sleep.

Took a nap before preparing a light supper. The dentist called around seven. Told him I had no pain or ill effects *after* the root canal. Also, how there was never numbness in my lip or jaw *during* the procedure.

He apologized for hurting me; and told me about his first root canal many years ago, during a period in dentistry when the minimizing of numbing agents was considered the best way to locate and remove the nerve. I appreciated his calling to check on me.

Thursday, May 22, 2008

After seeing an early client, answered my email, and ate lunch. While brushing my teeth, I noticed the area around last week's root canal site was red, swollen, and painful to the touch. Called my dentist who had me in the chair within the hour, installed an acrylic post to provide better anchorage for my over-bridge. Although this caused additional trauma to the already-inflamed tissue, the purpose is to keep food from getting stuck along the gumline. Not easy to eat with a sore mouth. He directed me to wear the bridge appliance as little as possible and to rinse frequently with salt water.

This will keep me from going out until the weekend, since the teeth involved are front and center. I'm relieved to have some down time. Saturday afternoon will end the dental quarantine.

Saturday, May 24, 2008

Cooked cereal for breakfast, and an egg. Have to chew slowly, since my bite on the left side is temporarily uneven. The right side provides only a tiny area of contact until the appliance adjusts.

Yesterday, overheard a discussion about a woman with scleroderma who is considering having all her teeth pulled. I wonder if pain or the frequent necessity for dental work will influence her decision. Expense could be a factor. Root canals and implants represent a substantial economic investment. Implants are not covered by dental insurance. Maybe this woman is simply looking to put an end to her ongoing mouth and gum problems.

Trying to keep as close as possible to my original smile and bite is a challenge. Motivation to keep my teeth is partly cosmetic; however, being better able to chew and digest my food is primary.

When my eldest grandchild was six, she warned me: "People who chew slowly live longer than people who chew fast." I bet her Japanese grandmother, or great grandmother, told her this. Sounds like a wise elder's cautionary tale.

Tuesday, May 27, 2008

I'm most relaxed when I eat alone, listening to NPR or reading the paper. Feel pressured in company, except when I'm with Bob or Nathalie who are slow eaters like me.

Thursday, September 18, 2008

Saw the dental hygienist early today. Over decades of quarterly cleanings, this was the first time with no tartar buildup. For all my brushing, flossing, rinsing and poking about with special picks, I'd never been able to halt the speedy formation of this veritable concrete wall between gums and teeth.

The phenomenon of a body becoming healthier—able to improve after fifty, whether the teeth, gums, or any other part— amazes me. When I consider I may have had scleroderma for almost than half a century, even this minor improvement in dental health seems miraculous.

Monday, October 13, 2008

Last night's party was great. I ate in slow bites, including dessert. Real strawberry shortcake's hard to pass up. Woke up during the wee hours with a twitch in my lower lip. Right away I began to wonder. Could this be a reaction to wearing the new night guard? The night guard designed to protect my lower permanent bridgework from being struck from above by the titanium implant post during sleep. As usual, my dentist was quick to respond.

He thought the twitch was probably from the way I was sleeping on my cheek, especially if my hand was underneath. His scarier suggestion: the twitch could be a symptom of blood vessel thinning from scleroderma with subsequent plugging of an important route from the side of my cheek, which he identified as the *mental nerve*. Inspired to take the best care of myself, I cancelled my afternoon clients.

Called Nathalie late in the afternoon; she got me laughing so hard I could feel the twitch beginning to loosen. By evening, the twitch was gone. I moved from fear to release to gratitude in the course of a few hours. Everyone ought to have a childhood friend, and access to the healing laughter, which began for us when we were eight and continues on. How better to encourage the expansion of a blood vessel!

SELF-CARE OPTIONS

Cleaning

If there is no soreness or other current teeth or gum problems, I brush after every meal with a good quality electric toothbrush. The cheaper battery brushes have a shorter span of usefulness and are practical when traveling.

For some, like me, who may react to mint flavoring, natural-flavored toothpastes are available in large grocery and health food stores. Among my favorites is fennel, a slight licorice flavor derived from a stalk plant.

When bridgework or implant anchors complicate cleaning, using a child's toothbrush around isolated tooth roots and implant structures works well. Tooth roots are teeth which have been ground down to accommodate special bridge work and are protected by a metal, or gold coverings, called copings, at the base; copings are not easy to keep clean and free from plaque. Brushing with a little baking soda early in the day may help. Because of the sodium content, baking soda brushing is not recommended for those with dry mouth or dry eye symptoms.

Water irrigation devices are good for washing small particles of food that brushing doesn't reach. Fluoride gel, if tolerated and doesn't cause GERD, can help protect against decay. Children's fluoride liquid rinses also come in flavors other than mint. However, some naturopathic doctors caution people with autoimmune diseases against the use of fluoride.

Those little pointed stimulators for cleaning between teeth are useful for getting at tiny pieces of nuts or seeds that elude brushes. This, and flossing, is easy to fit in during an evening's reading or TV-watching. My dentist recently suggested pipe cleaners, yes, pipe cleaners, for massaging and cleaning the area around isolated teeth and tooth roots.

A word of caution: New self-care disciplines are best introduced gradually, after consultation with dentist or hygienist. Overly rigorous brushing or stimulating may cause irritation or infection, and may cause damage to teeth and gums.

Smoking

Avoid cigarette and cigar smoking, as well as refined sugars in foods and in drinks.

ESOPHAGUS AND STOMACH

> "But I think there is genuine joy, too, a sense that no matter what, even if my stomach's growling, I'm going to dance. That's what I want to leave people with at the end of the play. After all this, people still know how to live."
>
> ~Jessica Hagedorn, actress

Jaw muscles and teeth coordinate in chewing. Then our swallowing muscles come into play. These muscles are both voluntarily and involuntarily controlled. Our will is active in the initial process of swallowing after which smooth muscle takes over.

Broken up food mixed with saliva or beverage travels down through the esophagus. Gravity helps, but the involuntary smooth muscle assists in moving the chewed food downward. If the esophagus has been damaged by acid splashing up from the stomach, a narrowing or stricture or ulcer may develop, slowing down or temporarily stopping the passage of food. Coughing or vomiting up stuck food or medication may bring temporary relief. However, informing your doctor at the first sign of any difficulty in swallowing, or when food or pills repeatedly get stuck en route, is imperative.

At the entrance to the stomach, there is a kind of door that is called the esophageal or gastro-esophageal junction. This door is designed to open only with swallowing, so that strong stomach acid, which serves to aid digestion and kill viruses, cannot splash back up and harm the esophagus. Stomach acid can travel upward as far as the mouth, resulting in a bitter taste, sore throat, and bad breath, especially noticeable in the morning after waking.

What is commonly called GERD, heartburn, or reflux, can seem to be nearly constant for persons with systemic scleroderma. In some cases this irritation causes cellular changes, which may lead to *Barrett's syndrome*, a precursor of cancer of the esophagus. In an effort to protect the esophagus, drugs called proton pump inhibitors (PPIs) are prescribed to inhibit the formation of stomach acid. Drugs called H2 blockers also may be recommended to help neutralize acidity.

Since smooth muscle lines the entire intestinal tract, functioning of the body's smooth muscle is at risk for hardening from overproduction of collagen in persons with SSc. The stomach may become slow to empty. This can bring about a feeling of nausea. Where serious destruction of the digestive tract has occurred, tube or IV feeding may be necessary.

A not-so-rare condition in scleroderma is commonly referred to as *watermelon stomach*. This name comes from the stripe-like appearance of dilated blood vessels on the stomach's inner lining. These vessels may bleed slightly and, over long periods, may cause anemia. Diet changes, drugs, laser treatment of bleeding points, and/or surgery are among the available therapies.

Wednesday, May 7, 2008

Arrived at The Center for Rheumatology a few minutes before nine, coughing a lot. My specialist said I was aspirating, inhaling tiny bits of food and saliva. Guess I was generating more stomach acid than I realized.

My errors in judgment began long before this morning; they began in the planning. I'd asked for an early appointment because earlier was more convenient for my friend Barbara who needed to get back by midafternoon. I hadn't felt like eating at 5:00 a.m., so hadn't taken my PPI. Worse came to worse.

Thursday, May 8, 2008

Having trouble swallowing my capsules. Since this happened several years back, I suspect my esophagus has narrowed and I'll require stretching during an endoscope procedure.

Thursday, June 5, 2008

A terrible weakness came over me this morning. Don't know why, since I'd slept well, finished work on Sunday's service, and had a fine breakfast. In the pool, coughed so much from aspirating, an RN in our swim group asked if I was okay. Had to stay upright treading water or else swim on my left side. Resting on the left side in bed is supposed to be help with reflux; so tried to translate the left-reclining posture to the water. After showering and oiling my body, came upstairs to lie down.

Sunday, June 30, 2008

A neighbor showed up in the exercise room with a CD of Mendelssohn's "Scottish Symphony" and walked to the music on the clonking treadmill alongside my stationary bike. Was already feeling sick from eating a handful of raisins too fast. They stayed stuck between throat and stomach. After going upstairs, I was able to throw them up without disturbing the supper that preceded them.

Thursday, August 8, 2008

There's definitely something wrong with my GI tract. A hiatal hernia complicates my situation even more. Can I skip days or a week of my PPIs without endangering my esophagus? Something's causing extreme irritation. I've developed reactions to most drugs after taking them for a while. I don't know what this is or what to do. Trying to avoid all spices, I'm worried about stomach acid splashing up while I'm sleeping, especially if I skip a PPI dosage.

Monday, August 11, 2008

I've only tomorrow to pack for the shore. After a full load of clients, made some visits to parishioners in nursing homes. Came back to swim and eat. Tiredness makes digestive problems worse. Took a little baking soda in water before sleep, but very drying to the mouth.

Friday, August 15, 2008

Tough getting to sleep after the family reunion dinner. My stomach's way off. Can't be the food. I chose well: broiled trout, salad, and mashed potatoes, and drank only Italian spring water.

Monday, August 18, 2008

Took 30 mgs. of my PPI several days ago thinking I'd be able to eat more at the reunion dinner. Still wasn't hungry; gave half my trout filet to a cousin. H2 blockers helped a little. I'm more sensitive to situations of stress these days; stomach churns when I'm tired or jumpy. Maybe I'm upset about losing my church job.

Sunday, August 24, 2008

Last night, couldn't eat, period. A couple of mouthfuls of leftover stir-fry came back up right away. Something got stuck halfway down. Kept trying, finger down throat, to bring it up. An hour later, I tried eating a small slice of watermelon, which also came up right away. After another hour or so of misery, I called my chiropractor who suggested I slowly sip an ounce or two of sparkling water. Happened to have a bottle of imported mineral water on hand. The first sip felt like a knife poking into my sternum, I wanted to throw up. Instead, I made myself wait, walked around, lifted my arms, twisted my torso, even attempted to jump up and down a few times, trying to get the swallow to go down all the way, which finally happened. If this is a stricture or narrowing of the esophagus, the sensation and symptoms are quite different from three years ago. I probably should make an appointment with the GI doctor. None of my physicians or practitioners suggested I do so, and I've told all of them about the problem.

This morning, thankful for eight hours of sleep, I cooked a multi-grain cereal thoroughly, but the graininess put me off. Weak and hungry, I scrambled an egg, toasted a piece of roll, and poured a cup of raspberry green tea. I chewed and swallowed everything carefully. A better start to a better day.

Wednesday, August 27, 2008

Been taking 15 mgs. of my PPI every morning; and no digestive problems since Sunday. Also, adding a teaspoon of aloe filet to my water bottle and chewing a little dried papaya after meals seems to help. Trying one thing after another, though I fear the problem is too complicated to solve on my own.

Friday, August 29, 2008

Thinking this morning about my gastro-intestinal history. Don't remember much before we moved to the country where at age nine I discovered there were foods I liked and foods I disliked. Evenings, after my sister and I did the dishes, I recall going upstairs to our room and lying face down on my bed with a pillow under my stomachache. During summers in Maine, we sometimes had lobster up to four times a week, steamed, or in salad or stew. Hot dogs, fried clams, and homemade French fries, I ate them all with as much gusto as any kid lucky enough to be there.

Saturday, August 30, 2008

GI tract behaving a little better. Trying to eliminate spices, especially garlic, almost an act of sacrilege to someone half Italian. Trying to plan meals around more alkaline foods. Tonight I had a yam, plain kidney beans with a little salt, and a mild sweet sausage. Unappetizingly Spartan.

Sunday, August 31, 2008

Life is changing fast. There's less excuse for the continuation of stressful work, spicy foods, or refined sugars. Letting the church job go, along with my beloved garlic and onions, not to speak of those moist dark brownies that appear during the congregation's fellowship hour, feels, on the one hand, like a sacrifice. On the other, the beginning satisfaction that I may be on the right path.

Tuesday, September 16, 2008

My chiropractor taught me a manipulation today for relieving GERD. I was leaning back on the treatment table when he pressed his fingers firmly into my sternum, with a downward pull toward my stomach. The spot was so tender; I drew back in a strong reflexive reaction. He said he uses this technique on himself to relieve reflux. I experimented later on, applying much less pressure, more like a gentle massage. The purpose is to relieve spasm of the esophagus and soothe the diaphragm. My massage version, before I go to bed, brings up gas suspended above my stomach and releases the tight, uncomfortable feeling in my upper abdomen.

Tuesday, September 23, 2008

This has been the worst day for my upper GI tract. Growing more concerned about the underlying reason.

Scheduled client appointments filled my planner until after seven last night. First mistake of the day was eating a bowl of a crunchy new cereal. A calcium capsule got stuck halfway down in esophageal limbo. Took a long a time to throw up the pills without losing the breakfast under them. All this left me shaky enough to doubt whether or not I would be able to carry out the day's schedule, including a late lunch with Bob.

Took a probiotic yogurt to the counseling office for my break. By 3:00, I had had some sunshine and rest, but nothing except the yogurt to eat. I took 150 milligrams of an H2 blocker toward the beginning of the meal, and had salad, beets, pasta, cooked greens, tiny bits of beef and chicken, even some dessert, which kept me going for the rest of the day. Realize this is no solution to the GERD problem or whatever else is happening on the way to my stomach. Right now, my doctors think going back on the PPI will solve everything. Frankly, as the one who owns this body, there is no difference whether I take the drug or not. I'm just as miserable either way.

Thursday, September 25, 2008

Determining what adversely affects breathing and swallowing is my ongoing continuing education project. Just now, after an apparently well-digested supper, I decided to try rinsing with a new mouthwash. After swooshing the mint-flavored antiseptic around in my mouth, the nausea, gassiness, there came the beginning of GERD. Tried to flush out the taste with water, but the mint continued to sting my throat and esophagus.

Mint tea's long been a problem, but never mouthwash. Since childhood, a blob of mint jelly on my plate alongside a lamb chop has felt fine. I did not swallow any of the mouthwash, so my reaction seemed extreme. As soon as I washed away the mint flavor with baking soda and water, I began to feel better. Sipped a little baking soda and water for good measure. Here's the thing: maybe I have had a reaction to mint toothpaste and/or mouthwash and ignored it, or chalked it up to indigestion. Lately, I'm more aware of how I feel after tasting than ever before. This hypersensitivity's annoying and helpful at the same time. I can see why so many people are willing to continue to take acid-reducing drugs even when they cause uncomfortable side effects. Much easier than trying to develop a discipline of nearly constant vigilance. So far, nearly constant vigilance hasn't worked for me.

Tuesday, September 30, 2008

When I get too hungry, the way I choose, chew, swallow, and digest food is influenced more by emotions than by my body's need; today's behavior was plain crazy. I'd been practicing, and then singing for the High Holy Days for about five hours. On meeting Bob for a late lunch at a restaurant chain, I imagined, since I'd taken 30 mgs. of the PPI, I could down a burger with mushrooms, Swiss cheese and bacon, French fries, cold slaw, and cottage cheese. I recognized my selection as a mad assumption even before ordering, but undifferentiated hunger blinded and compelled me. Only the cottage cheese was easy. Just the sight of the stuffed burger had a monstrous impact. I felt nauseated before the first mouthful. After my terror subsided, I calmed down and ate most everything on my plate with no immediate consequences. Persistent in excess, I grabbed a handful of dark chocolate wafers and a glass of milk at Bob's house before driving home.

A nap, a light supper, a workout, and here I am at the start of the Hebrew peoples' Days of Awe, certain before morning I'll suffer for my gastronomical sins.

Wednesday, October 1, 2008

Hard to admit I goofed again after yesterday's defeat. Back from the out-of-town staff meeting, I went with Bob to a diner where I indulged in gravy and other acidic stuff. In the pool an hour later, heartburn was so bad I couldn't swim at all, at least not horizontally. Stayed upright in the water, clinging with my feet along the edge where the pool floor bows to meet the wall. No matter how well covered by drug therapy, I cannot eat without thinking.

Sunday, October 5, 2008

This morning at breakfast, listening to music on NPR, I wondered if I might find a way to make swallowing capsule supplements easier. I prefer capsules to pills because they're soft and slippery instead of hard and chalky. No matter, whichever one gets stuck partway down, there's a painful dilemma: Should I try to retrieve with finger down throat? An attempt to push the capsule on with more water hurts, while throwing up sours my stomach for hours. I'd begun to assign traumatic association to swallowing all capsules, which was leading to further tightening of my throat.

At first, I tried to solve the problem by taking huge gulps of water with each capsule. This method traps air in my esophagus, which takes effort to burp up and makes aspiration more likely. My impatience with having to burp up air often caused the capsule to remain stuck for a longer time. (My grandson thinks being able to burp up air intentionally is a thrilling sport.) Pouring more water on top of the capsule is like jumping from a stream into the ocean.

Technique: I put a capsule on the center of my tongue and drawing most of the air out of my mouth so that the capsule was tightly surrounded by my inner cheek and tongue. Took a glass of room-temperature water and drew in a small stream, just enough to swallow the pill, while slightly tucking in my chin. The tucked chin is a posture to ease swallowing. With this method, the capsule went right down. Another sip sealed the deal. Even when I'm hurried, this usually works; being unhurried works better.

Wednesday, October 22, 2008

Just read in *The Scleroderma Exchange* about the benefits of eating smaller, more frequent meals. For one, the stomach has a chance to empty more quickly. At my fifth small meal of the day, I took a thimbleful of mint jelly with my lamb chops. Throat closed right away. Later, gave into another bad impulse. Shortly before turning in, I scarfed down some almond butter on crackers. In the same way that almond butter sticks like glue to a knife, the almond butter stuck to the lining of my esophagus. Tortuously, slowly, I removed the glue with licorice-tinted chamomile tea. For people with esophageal issues, no snack before bedtime is the rule.

December 3, Wednesday, 2008

Composed my end-of-year report at 6:00 a.m. with copies for the counseling center's board and staff, etc. Had trouble with my grain drink coffee substitute; threw it up after downing only half a cup. Maybe the barley's the culprit. I can't recall having trouble with the drink in the past.

Friday, December 12, 2008

Whenever I eat with people at a dinner party, I get tense, afraid I'll delay the next course. I can't eat fast.

Monday, December 22, 2008

Christmas is shaping up to be a two-dinner day. Bob's daughter from Vermont and her daughter, as well as two of her sons will be arriving from afar. Our estimated convergence time is 7:00 p.m., rather late to feast. The first dinner has been set for 2:00 p.m. when local family will gather. During the interval before the next party, we can go back to our respective homes to rest. The late-arriving younger crowd should have no problem with gravy before bed.

Monday, January 19, 2009

Back from errands, made a chicken stew. Funny thing was I couldn't eat the chicken, only the broth and vegetables. Reflux after supper seemed to come from swallowing several capsules too close together. I had trouble getting them down, even with my new pill-swallowing technique.

Sunday, February 1, 2009

I deserve to suffer after pushing myself to go out this morning. Ate lunch too fast and ended up taking an H2 blocker. Have to get over thinking I can eat automatically like the millions of people who salivate, chew, and swallow an unexamined variety of foodstuffs with no apparent ill effects.

Saturday, February 7, 2009

Have to wait a few weeks for my appointment with the GI doctor. Until diagnosed, I'm following some of Cayce's remedies for scleroderma sufferers. I went to the store and shopped for vegetables to make his all-vegetable soup, a recipe I found on the Internet. "Don't cook the vegetables with meat" directive about making Cayce's all-vegetable soup. Bought a piece of beef round from which to make "beef juice," another of Casey's elixirs. This requires a few pounds piece of fresh raw beef. Following the directions from memory, I put the meat into a dry saucepan with a tight lid. The sauce pan holding the beef I placed into a larger pot containing enough water to simmer around the outside of the smaller pan. Occasionally had to add water to the outer pot. After several hours of simmering, the pot with the piece of beef inside contained about two cups of the rich and satisfying "juice" or broth. The meat itself became like a piece of old leather, fit to be thrown away, or given to a dog keen on the challenge of the chew.

Wednesday, February 18, 2009

After a good sleep, was surprised to have digestive trouble again. Breakfast of fruit, yogurt, and whey protein before swimming seemed to go down fine. When I came upstairs for my second small breakfast and vitamins, I had terrible reflux. Not even a cup of chamomile tea helped. The teaspoon of omega-3 oil finished me off. Selective vomiting got up the oil and the calcium capsule with a large amount of mucus.

Thursday, February 19, 2009

At first I thought I'd been given an intestinal bug for my birthday. Saw two clients this morning even though I felt crappy. Was feverish by noon. The face staring back at me from the mirror looked sunburned. By the time I sat down to an early lunch of fresh boiled asparagus and a tiny bowl of warmed beef juice, I realized to go out with friends tonight would be crazy. Couldn't get down even a few forkfuls. Called the couple who had planned to join us and cancelled.

My birthday celebration turned out to consist of cheery emails from my son and grandson, and a bouquet of telephone greetings. Spoke end to end with Nathalie, Barbara, and Bob while snug under the covers; watched TV and slept. Scleroderma-related illnesses always bring on a certain amount of fear; and this is no virus.

Tuesday, February 24, 2009

Up and fully dressed before 6:00 a.m., read a Psalm, exercised, and considered the coming of Lent. Tomorrow is Ash Wednesday. Mortality's uppermost in my mind this year. After a bowl of cereal, I made the mistake of trying to swallow a calcium capsule which got stuck midway down. Saw the nurse practitioner at the GI office who set me up for the endoscope procedure. She says dilation will solve the problem.

Thursday, February 26, 2009

An early morning appointment with my local rheumatologist. Aside from what he agrees looks like a need for esophageal dilation, apparently, I'm doing fine.

He said esophageal narrowing or stricture is not necessarily scleroderma-related, that lots of people have it in later life. Is this part of getting older? He found only minute fluid retention in my right knee, fingers less swollen from sclerodactyly than in previous years, heart and lungs okay, no shortness of breath while exercising.

I'm experiencing a little mania from this cluster of doctors' visits. At lunch with Bob today, began to debate whether or not I really need the gastro-endoscope procedure after all. I'd like to forget the whole thing.

Saturday, February 28, 2009

How strange life is. Much of the time I would like to dedicate myself to some altruistic good in hope of alleviating some pain in the world. For most of humanity, the Lenten theme of loss, of inwardness, does not pass with the season. There's also an undeniable side of me that would like to be free, to enjoy some useless pleasure.

A few days ago, on Fat Tuesday, the day of feasting before the attitude of fasting, I took an unopened bottle of gift wine to a friend downstairs, someone whose apartment, unlike mine, contains a corkscrew. We drank a glass together and afterwards finished off a bowl of chocolate pudding. There were these marvelous moments when I was completely relaxed, a little high, the way people who don't have digestive ills are free to be.

Wednesday, March 4, 2009

This is the day of my esophageal procedure. The GI specialist went light on the twilight sleep anesthetic, as I asked. While the attendant wheeled me back to the cubicle where Bob was waiting, my question was: "Are you taking me to another room for the procedure?"

"You've already had the procedure," she answered.

I had to ask the same question again because there was no pain or other evidence of the invasion, no dizziness, no discomfort anywhere in my body. The invasion of which I had been so wary was a piece of cake. On the other hand, as I quickly learned, the doctor found a large ulcer at the base of my esophagus. No narrowing, no stricture, is the good news. The ulcer, photographed in living color, is the bad news. The doctor pointed out mine exceeds the 1-4 scale. Clearly, my number-5 ulcer was oozing blood and blocking entry to my stomach.

The drug prescribed by my GI doctor for treatment happens to be the same proton pump inhibitor that I rejected a few years back when I was experimenting to find a PPI I could tolerate. Now I'm directed to take 40 milligrams a half hour before breakfast and 40 a half hour before supper, an industrial-strength dosage for my reed-like frame. The drug scares me as much as the ulcer itself. Nevertheless, I intend to proceed with a kill-or-cure attitude.

After my first pill, I felt a sensation like my throat closing off. Bob came right over. After a couple of hours, felt better and finally went to bed with a castor oil pack (and a prayer) over my sternum. Before sleep, I swallowed two teaspoons of something called a suspension drug to coat the esophageal lining overnight, after which I felt almost as bad as before.

During all those months, while I complained about having trouble swallowing, not one of my physicians thought to warn me that my esophagus may in trouble. Told each of my doctors and other practitioners about the capsules, about food getting stuck midway, about the pain and the vomiting; and not one of them advised me to make an appointment with the GI doctor, and to begin lobbying for this essential diagnostic procedure. I came to this conclusion after almost a year of experimenting with my own lame solutions.

Ergo: I am the one, as my own caretaker, whose responsibility it is not only to initiate but to approach the medical system assertively, if necessary, about persistent pain or dysfunction. That was and is not an easy thing to do.

My job now is to foster healing of the ulcer. When I asked my GI specialist about the cells he took for biopsy, he said they looked okay, and he could let me know for sure in a couple of weeks.

Thursday, March 5, 2009

My stomach feels peculiar after meds and an early breakfast. Could the weakness and pain be from the heavy-duty PPI? These are two of the side effects listed on the accompanying printout. Would I feel better if I hadn't read the printout?

Midmorning, my second meal, apple, banana, whey protein, and probiotic yogurt went into the blender. I took the suspension drug. Small meal, I thought; yogurt digests itself; and I am staying true to my prescribed meds. The drink was on the table near the computer. I began to sip while answering emails. All of a sudden, my throat began to tighten; my ears felt hot and swollen. I called the druggist who told me if I have any trouble breathing to call 911, to call my doctor, too. I'm reluctant to contact the GI specialist's office; he may think I'm rejecting his treatment.

Friday, March 6, 2009

Up in the wee hours writing a fax to the GI doc asking for a substitution for either the suspension drug or the PPI, whichever one he suspects may be the cause of the throat tightening.

After the biggest breakfast I could manage, I went to the pool. Was shaky and weak after swimming. The GI nurse called me back to say people rarely react to the PPI medication or suspension drug, and to keep on taking them.

Translation: "It's all in your head."

Called my internist, thinking maybe he could unravel my symptoms. If they are coming from the ulcer itself, why were they so much milder before the procedure than they are now?

My internist came up with a pretty good theory: Since the suspension drug is designed to bond with protein, an esophageal spasm may have occurred due to the condensed protein in the whey drink. Giving up the whey protein may be the answer. Whey is also a cow milk product. Maybe I'm lactose intolerant like my mother.

Lunch was difficult. After two hours I got under the covers but couldn't sleep. Tonight Bob and I planned to eat out with friends. They made the hour early to accommodate my schedule. Took the new PPI and the suspension drug and was intentional about having an enjoyable time. At the buffet, I chose from a variety of dishes, but my appetite was small and the array of choices suddenly unappealing. About an hour after taking my meds, I got that sensation again, like two hands squeezing my throat. This occurred while telling stories and laughing with friends, so I know that my reaction was not the result of anxiety, or whey.

Back home, dialed my insurance company's on-call nurse who helped me organize questions for on-call doctor. Inconveniently for me, perhaps conveniently for him, my GI specialist is on vacation this week.

Applied a castor oil pack to my sternum for about a half hour, remembering Edgar Cayce's admonishment about carrying out therapies with spiritual intention. As I felt the warm weight of the hot water bottle's pressure over the "pack," I asked for healthy new tissue to replace that which is diseased and inflamed.

Saturday, March 7, 2009

Up at 5:00, lips swollen. There's tingling in my fingers; they're puffy, sausage-like, as they haven't been in years. Mouth's dry; and I'm having trouble swallowing. I'm scared. How will I be able to eat? The way to figure out if this is drug-related is to eliminate one or the other of the drugs for a day or two. The GI physician on call suggested I try going off the suspension drug first.

A long massage this afternoon relaxed me. Good conversation with the therapist. Laughed a few times, which felt great. I came home to eat my fish and noodles in silent dread. I'm afraid of my medications; I'm afraid of my food. Even noodles, which are my favorite, under suspicion.

About an hour before bedtime, felt the weird tightness in my ears and throat again. Who can I call? I'm not in a good negotiating place with the medical team. My GI specialist isn't back yet; and his nurse is annoyed with me. Easy to get a little paranoid when I don't know what's going on in my body.

Sunday, March 8, 2009

The GI nurse was abrupt in answering my questions last Friday. She referred me back to my internist. She doesn't want to get in the middle of a controversy about drug reactions. Made an appointment with my internist for later in the week.

Tuesday, March 10, 2009

Back from my office, I went online to research ulcer diets. There's conflict in cyberspace about what does and what does not work. For GERD, eat at an apple; don't eat an apple. Low fiber is recommended for ulcers, with an allowance for cooked brown rice and low-acid vegetables. The other allowable fruits are ripe bananas, mangos, and melons.

I'm going to read the jokes in *The New Yorker* then apply a castor oil pack, hoping to sleep better than last night.

Wednesday, March 11, 2009

Friend Barbara, always a sign of high energy and true love, woke me up last night from a sound asleep with a brainstorm. She said if I could be hospitalized to deal with the side effects from the prescribed drugs, the trouble and expense may be worth the trouble. Afterwards, I lay there thinking. With a little help from my friends, I could "hospitalize" myself, that is: stay in, rest, and eat only the simplest food, eliminate stress, and build strength. Way before dawn, I'm already planning to cancel most of my clients for the rest of the week, to arrange for my virtual "hospitalization."

By 5:00 p.m. I felt starved. A big bowl of artichoke hearts and tofu over rice, a grilled cheese sandwich, and the rest of Cayce's beef juice, disappeared at one sitting. I fell upon my food like a wild animal, hardly tasting or chewing. I'd do well with a dietitian to help me through this week of "hospitalizing" myself.

Friday, March 13, 2009

My supervisor and I spoke by phone this afternoon. Beyond a brief discussion of clients and treatment plans, speaking with him put me in touch with the special loneliness of being ill. The same loneliness I felt as a child of five when, boarded in a convent orphanage, I was confounded by my caretakers who spoke mostly French.

Sunday, March 15, 2009

This Sabbath day is bright. Had a great sleep with less dryness in my throat and mouth. After Madrigal rehearsal, I went for my first swim since the procedure. Pool seemed cooler than usual. The tips of my fingers turned blue.

My internist called. He tried to convince me that the GI specialist would not be mad at me for taking a drug other than the one he prescribed, since all of these acid-reducing drugs are designed to do the same thing.

Monday, March 16, 2009

Before I can sing tonight's rehearsal, I'll need a nap and a well-digested meal.

The GI doc called at 5:00 p.m. He asked kindly about my "many questions." He said the feelings of weakness and other symptoms I've been experiencing are not related to the medications at all, but to the ulcer. As for the biopsy, the cells on the surface of the ulcer were normal, showing no signs of *Barrett's Syndrome*. He said to make an appointment early in April for another endoscope procedure, so that he can evaluate the degree of healing, and take a biopsy of the cells underneath the ulcer site.

Toward the end of our conversation, he made me laugh. He said having a glass of wine or beer occasion would be all right. I've avoided drinking for years, but his suggestion freed me to dig fearlessly into one of the pork chops I'd cooked for Bob's dinner. Minutes before he called, I'd been thinking how good they looked.

In our telephone conversation, the doctor cited loose clothing, a raised bed at night and medication as most effective in maintaining esophageal health. Diet, he said, is the least-effective tool in managing reflux. Even if eating particular foods might contribute in the smallest way to my healing, I intend to keep searching to discover what they might be.

Tuesday, March 17, 2009

Early this morning I emailed a medical update to my Albany rheumatologist. He answered a predictable "yes" to my question about whether the esophageal ulcer is related to having scleroderma.

An amazingly nice day, warmest so far this year. Before my 3:00 appointment, I sat for a half hour on a bench outside the church building facing into the sun, sleeves rolled up. Worked out after supper, and am about to wind down and get into bed. My night off from applying the castor oil pack. I've been faithful with both the oil and the prayer. Thankful for today's gift of sunshine.

Wednesday, March 18, 2009

Dragged myself out of bed for 7:30 healing service. After a late breakfast, I bought a pair of sorry gray slacks with the essential elastic around the waist at a neighborhood thrift shop, and a choke-less, mango-colored turtleneck. I'm reassured to find clothes kinder to my esophageal pathway. To find clothes kinder to my aesthetics is my next goal. Later, in a department store's intimate apparel section, I was transformed from queen of the underwire uplift to sports-bra matron. I'm willing to be flatter and lower in exchange for having nothing poking into my sternum. Was never aware of the importance of non-restrictive clothing until the GI doc's warning.

Seems every time I close my eyes to meditate, I'm lying under layers of castor oil and moist wool, chin to chin with my old hot water bottle. In all seriousness, there may be no better place for prayer.

Friday, April 3, 2009

This morning was my second endoscope procedure. Afterwards, still in the treatment room, my GI doc announced the ulcer is 100 percent healed. Bob brought me home. Knelt by my bed awhile before climbing in to sleep the day away.

Saturday, April 18, 2009

A friend offered to drive me to a concert tonight. We got seats ticketed in the same row. Felt crappy, wanted to cancel, but didn't. Instead, took a couple of antihistamines, which suppressed my sneezing, runny nose, and itchy legs. Well worth the effort for the sake of *A German Requiem* by Brahms, especially those moments when the chorus and brass fall in love with each other. Best of all, the soprano's single aria, pure liquid gold, carried me high and away.

Tuesday, April 23, 2009

I first thought these symptoms were SSc-related. The excruciating itching I'd heard about? These are definitely allergy hives. Last time I had them this bad was in my twenties after a shot of penicillin.

When I called the druggist last night and told him about the lung congestion and hives, he said I could be reacting to any one of several drugs and to call my doctor, which I did. My internist said he'd stop by on his way to the hospital at 7:00 this morning to take a look. He doesn't make house calls, but the hospital is near my co-op, and we've been friends for years. He took me off all meds until the reaction subsides.

Saturday, May 2, 2009

Here I am at the mountaintop monastery hoping to find some direction about what to do next. What foods to eat? What medications to take? I'm drinking their mountain well water, which is out of this world.

SELF-CARE OPTIONS

Applications: Castor Oil Pack

Castor Oil, derived from the castor bean, can be bought in health food stores in various quantities. Some brands will have instructions for Edgar Cayce's "castor oil pack" printed on the bottle's label. He recommended the "pack" for healing as well as for maintenance of gastro-intestinal health. For persons with scleroderma, Cayce directed that both abdomen and back, over the kidney area, be the focus of treatments. See instructions in the Glossary for making a castor oil pack.

Castor oil in drugstores tends to be packaged in small bottles and is expensive, harkening back to the days when taking castor oil internally was a common remedy for constipation.

Clothing

Tight jeans, skirts with belts, and binding undergarments can seriously interfere with the digestive process. In women, the area most likely to be pinched or cramped is between esophagus and stomach. Men's clothing tends toward adjustable belts and waistbands.

For women, stylish slacks and jeans with elastic or expandable waists come in every size and length, and are available to order from casual catalogues. Buying one size larger in stretch slacks or jean styles with a slightly below-the-waist closing, will fit well over the buttocks and provide a couple of inches around the waist for soft belting, or for threading of elastic in the waistband. The ideal bra has good uplift with no wires. Most department stores have staff experienced in helping customers find the best style and fit.

Foods

Consultation with a good dietitian, nutritionist, or naturopathic doctor may be helpful in finding the foods and supplements for one's particular needs. These practitioners should have some understanding of gastrointestinal issues in SSc.

There is information on the Internet, encouraging persons with autoimmune diseases to change to a gluten-free diet. This is not easy to accomplish and may be unnecessary for certain individuals. In Europe, there are special provisions in the healthcare system for persons diagnosed with celiac disease, and for whom a gluten-free diet is prescribed. In the U.S, celiac disease is less familiar to general practitioners; and most have no awareness that celiac disease and sensitivity to gluten are more common in persons with SSc than in the general population. Neither may be definitively diagnosed from a routine blood test. An endoscope procedure is believed to deliver a more reliable diagnosis.

Some foods may lead to a slightly more alkaline balance in the body which some believe can improve digestive and general health. Chiropractic physician, John O.A. Pagano, has done comprehensive research and writing about the acid/alkaline balance and recommends specific changes in diet and food combinations. He lists foods he has used in treatment with his own patients, and includes reference to scleroderma. His recommendations include a surprisingly large quantity of green vegetables to be eaten every day, as well as fruit, grains, lamb, poultry, and fish.

Dr. Pagano also points to specific chiropractic adjustments that may assist in the restoration, and/or maintenance of digestive health.

Refined sugars are acid-making machines. Sweeteners such as buckwheat honey, molasses, and real maple syrup may be used in minute quantities. They have some nutritional value and may be better tolerated than refined sugars. Popular artificial sweeteners may cause metabolic problems in certain people; they do in me.

Lactose intolerance is a common problem. One of the symptoms is diarrhea; the onset may be a few hours to a day after the ingestion of cow's milk, cheese, or ice cream. Plain yogurt, if tolerated, is beneficial to the GI tract. Some persons fare better with Greek or goat milk yogurt, both of which digest more readily than commercial cow-milk varieties. I often mix the plain organic yogurt with organic probiotic yogurt; the latter contains some sugar integral to its manufacture. Buttermilk is a cultured product that may be used, according to taste. First check the ingredients of certain brands for added "milk."

If taking protein drinks as a supplement, take caution. Whey is a derived milk product; watch out for lactose intolerance. Many people are allergic to soy. Even egg white protein may trigger a reaction in sensitive people. Probably the most easily tolerated booster supplement is rice protein. Even with this product, beware of a long list of amino acids on the label, as these, in greater quantities, may encourage weight loss. A further consideration: rice protein taken alone is an incomplete protein and requires combining with other foods to be utilized by the body for cell building and renewal.

Massage
This is a known stress reliever and increases circulation to and relaxation of connective tissue. Having the phone number of a licensed therapeutic massage therapist on hand when a relative asks about a holiday gift is a good

idea. Helpful self-massage before sleep may be done by massaging the fingers into the lower sternum area with a gentle downward motion.

Sleep: A Raised Bed

Sleeping on a bed four-to-six inches higher at the head than at the feet enlists gravity to help keep stomach acid from splashing upward. This incline is easiest for back sleepers. Side sleepers can end up with occasional spine or leg pain from the odd angle, even on firm memory foam mattresses. A quality spring mattress topped with a featherbed also can provide a comfortable pressure-free surface. Even for side sleepers, the upward incline is better than sleeping on a flat surface. To avoid reflux, lying on the left side is more effective than lying on the right. To facilitate stomach emptying, sleeping on the right side is better.

Spices

Omission of strong spices helps block GERD in many people. The vegetables, fruits, and spices with the worst reputation are black pepper, chili, garlic, onions, and wine vinegars, citrus fruits, with the exception of tangerines and fresh lemons. Red tomatoes, tomato paste and catsup may be especially disruptive because their acid content

Stress Avoidance

Whenever possible, eat in a quiet atmosphere. Be alert to the tone of conversation among friends and family. Better eat alone than where there is anger or dissent. Self-care includes avoiding toxic people as well as ingesting toxic substances.

Supplements

A natural protective coating for the esophagus and stomach may be found in DGL, deglycyrrhizinated licorice. Derived from licorice root, DGL is chemically altered to avoid causing a rise in blood pressure, as may unaltered licorice products. Chewable DGL, which contains no sugar or artificial sweeteners, is hard to find. There are, however, easy-to-swallow capsules that eliminate the sugar/sweetener issue. Contraindication warnings exist for women who are pregnant, or those using certain other herbals or medications. Your druggist and/or physician should be consulted about using this, as any other supplement.

Aloe filet, from the aloe plant, has known healing properties and is used both as application to the skin, and for soothing the digestive tract. Aloe filet is a good occasional addition to drinking water. A gelatinous liquid obtainable in health food stores, aloe has a slight lemony flavor. Check for contraindications.

Chamomile tea is a tried and true friend of the digestive tract. Adding a little apple juice to this tea increases its alkalinity. Ginger and turmeric are reportedly good for digestion. They can be used alone or together in very small amounts, steeped in hot water as teas, or added to soup and rice dishes. However, these are spices which, taken too frequently, or in excessive amounts, can further irritate an inflamed GI tract.

Upper-Body Exercise

Lifting weights requires informed instruction and/or supervision. This expands the muscles of the chest, and lifts the diaphragm, with the effect of lengthening and relaxing the esophageal area. Certain water exercises provide similar benefits.

Water and Other Beverages

Drinking a glass of spring water or other alkaline beverage, such as decaffeinated tea or broth, half an hour before a meal is beneficial; while drinking quantities of beverages with your meal may increase gas and bloating. Because I no longer drink wine, beer, sodas, or other processed beverages, I purchase bottled water from Italy, France, or New Zealand for an occasional treat.

Persons with scleroderma who suffer from dry mouth must sip water constantly in order to moisten and swallow their food. For those who do not have to sip a beverage while eating, digestion may be enhanced by taking liquid refreshment a while before, but not during, a meal. This is a tip borrowed from yoga lore.

Alcoholic and carbonated drinks stimulate acid production, as well as dehydrate and flood the digestive system with non-nutritive sugars or artificial sweeteners. Coffee is acidic and may lower blood sugar slightly and cause jumpiness in some people. For others, coffee is tolerable, even beneficial, if taken without cream or sugar. Edgar Cayce was a promoter of black coffee as a GI stimulant. Coffee and teas, other than chamomile or steeped fresh ginger, need to be tested for individual tolerance.

LOWER DIGESTIVE TRACT

"The tuba is the most intestinal of instruments, the very lower bowel of music."

~Peter De Vries

The lengthy small intestine is not accessible to gastro-endoscope procedures. Sometimes waste from the colon pushes up into the small intestine causing bacterial infection. If a portion of the intestine loses function from the hardening of smooth muscle, a serious condition called pseudo obstruction may occur. This is relatively uncommon in SSc and has few corrective solutions; there is, however, hope for future bowel transplantation procedures.

The bowels work best when sufficient fiber and water are consumed. Where there is destruction of smooth muscle, constipation may become a chronic problem. Bacterial overgrowth also may occur when movement of waste toward excretion is too slow. Antibiotics are generally prescribed for this condition, often in a series of treatments. Many people are helped by including probiotics in their diet from capsules or, better, from live yogurts, which contain bacteria that are friendly to the intestines and facilitate movement.

The likelihood of constipation increases when collagen formation hardens smooth muscle in the GI tract. Use of laxatives may temporarily enable bowel function; however, this does not solve the problem over time, and may even cause harm. Exercise, nutritive oils such as olive and almond, and fibers such as ground flaxseed and stewed prunes, as well as daily inclusion of fresh fruit and vegetables are often helpful in restoring normal function.

There is a greater chance of diarrhea as well as constipation in those with SSc. Medications and sensitivity to certain foods such as those containing milk or gluten, may contribute to diarrhea and/or weight loss. Checking thyroid function and blood sugar levels is essential, because having an autoimmune disease does not eliminate the possibility of acquiring other diseases or conditions. Malfunctioning of the thyroid gland or pancreas, for instance, can affect the manner in which nutrients are absorbed and waste excreted.

Many people with SSc develop a weakening of the anal sphincter. This can cause leakage requiring the wearing of a protective absorbent pad. This symptom may be intermittent and has been known to abate with exercise and/ or diet changes.

Over the last six years, I've had several bouts of constipation that did not respond to any of the recommended non-nutritive fiber supplements. The fiber mixtures worked for one or two days after which I became bloated without the action. As for laxatives, none of the many brands I tried, including one obtained by prescription, was effective for more than two days. Advice from a GI nurse practitioner to eat probiotic yogurt daily was the most helpful in the restoration of normal function.

Three years ago, after a colonoscopy with polyps removal, I was tested for food sensitivities by a nutritionist on the staff of a chiropractic practice. At the time I did not recognize the connection between my diet and bowel function. I had experienced chronic constipation for six months. Eating spouted wheat and prunes did not solve the problem. The nutritionist recommended I eliminate certain foods for a period of eight weeks. Her testing method seemed more intuitive than scientific. She recorded my muscle strength as I held and smelled vials containing various foods, sweeteners, and drugs. She nixed peanuts, chicken, cow dairy, oatmeal, and wheat products, among other foods common to my diet. After seeing my reaction to three sample PPIs, she identified the one I am best able to tolerate.

Concurrent with the nutritionist's recommendations, I began to take an herbal remedy containing plant tannis to treat what my former chiropractor suspected may be intestinal infection. I took the daily tannis capsule while following the new diet. In less than a week, my bowels began to move naturally. For two months I continued the tannis supplement, in an amount much lower than the dose first recommended, because of my initial reactivity. After I stopped taking the herbal and returned to my former diet, improvement in my lower bowel health held for about a year. Since the prescribed diet changes were concurrent with taking the herbal tannis, I could not determine if the diet or the plant tannis, the two together, or neither, led to my improved lower bowel health.

SELF-CARE OPTIONS

Exercise

Bike-riding, or rowing, on exercise machines or outdoors, encourages bowel motility. Energetic walking, working out with weights, laughing, and sexual release, all have their place in maintaining the natural rhythm of digestion and excretion.

Foods

The lower bowel usually responds to nutritive fiber. Plums, fresh, dried, or cooked into good old stewed prunes are a classic fiber source. Seeds and raisins, apples eaten separate from other foods with their skin, and sprouted grains also are on the list. Some gluten-sensitive persons can tolerate small amounts of sprouted wheat and other spouted grains. Whole grain cooked cereals, as well as brown rice, beans and lentils, all contain a powerhouse of fiber and nutrition, and usually contribute to lower bowel health. There are delicious gluten-free hot cereals including quinoa flakes, a seed derivative which is rich in easily digestible protein.

If you have a problem with chewing seeds, nuts, and apples, consider nut butters, especially almond, and tahini, which is basically sesame seeds and oil. Almonds are the most alkaline of nuts.

Probiotic yogurts have live bacteria able to survive the journey through the entire digestive tract into the colon, or lower bowel; they are effective in facilitating movement when eaten regularly. The Latin names for these bacteria are listed on the labels, and include acidophilus, bifidus and probiotic bifidobacterium lactis. Some popularly advertised probiotic yogurts contain more than seven percent sugar. Purer, plainer products may be found in large grocery or health food stores. Kefir or buttermilk usually will not disturb bowel function, unless lactose intolerance is severe.

Fresh vegetables, raw, steamed or boiled, are recommended in the amount of four to six servings a day. A serving is about a handful. Modest amounts of broiled fish, lamb, and poultry broiled or cooked in water with mild herbs or spices constitute nutritional variety and do not block normal intestinal function and excretion. These foods generally follow Edgar Cayce's guidelines for persons with scleroderma. Beef and shellfish are acidic and slow to digest.

When available and affordable, fresh local organically grown grains, produce, and grain-fed cage-free eggs are preferred over commercially farmed. Taste, freshness, and nutritional quality all might be considered in the choice of live foods.

Massage

Massage can be a helpful aid to motility in the lower GI tract. Several years ago, I went to a therapeutic massage practitioner to assist in breaking my pattern of constipation. After a few sessions, I asked about massaging myself. She advised me lie on my back and keep all hand motion and pressure going clockwise and circular, starting at the belly button, and moving only in a downward motion into and through the pelvic area.

Water and Hydration

Become a water connoisseur. Drink freely from the purest water you can find. Artesian well water is naturally alkaline and available in some health food stores. Filter tap water for drinking and cooking. Bottle water from approved spring or mountain sources. Glass containers are best for water storage.

Avoid plastic containers especially in summer. Carry water in ecology-safe, glass-lined bottles for sipping during the day and while traveling.

Chapter 4
LUNGS/HEART/KIDNEYS

"Who will tell whether one happy moment of love or the joy of breathing or walking on a bright morning and smelling the fresh air is not worth all the suffering and effort which life implies."

~Erich Fromm

LUNGS

Our lungs are designed to take oxygen from the air as we breathe in and release carbon dioxide waste as we breathe out. These twin organs have a sponge-like appearance. Near their center, bronchial tubes divide off from the windpipe and into numerous smaller branches that have clusters of alveoli at their tips. Alveoli are tiny, round air sacs. The walls, or membranes, that surround these air sacs must remain thin and flexible enough to permit the flow of oxygen into the capillaries within. In turn, red cells transport oxygen from these vessels to arteries which supply all the body's cells.

Capillaries are the smallest blood vessels. When oxygen flows to the capillaries and/or alveoli become blocked, oxygen levels in the blood drop. In the systemic forms of scleroderma, there may be narrowing or occlusion of some of these small blood vessels in the lungs. In addition, thickening from collagen of the air sac's normally paper-thin membrane may diminish oxygen flow to the capillaries.

Reflux may contribute to fibrosis, or hardening of lung tissue, because inflammation of the alveoli can develop from the involuntary spillage of stomach acid into the airway. In individuals with scleroderma, this occurs if the valve at the bottom of the esophagus is too weak to prevent the upward flow of gastric acid; and too weak to quickly clear it. The frequently prescribed proton pump inhibitors (PPIs) reduce the production of stomach acids but do not prevent reflux. When reflux is severe, the esophagus and the airways are exposed to the injurious effects of stomach contents.

Pulmonary arterial hypertension (PAH) occurs in this illness when where there is high resistance to the flow of blood through the lungs to pick up oxygen, so less oxygen reaches the organs and limbs. There are procedures and laboratory tests to help detect the presence of PAH. Persons at risk of developing pulmonary hypertension should be tested annually. The first year's tests provide a baseline for comparison with future tests.

Ever since the year I was diagnosed with SSc, I have had annual pulmonary function and six-minute walk tests, as well as echocardiograms. Although I have symptoms indicating PAH, my case is considered mild. Breathlessness with exertion, which was frequent in my thirties and a characteristic symptom of PAH, is not one of my symptoms at present.

Changes in test results, along with worsening symptoms, may indicate a need for referral to a pulmonary or cardiology specialist. Finding a doctor who has had experience in treating persons with SSc is important. The specialist will monitor your condition over time, and may recommend a right heart catheterization, which is essential for making a definitive diagnosis of PAH. The physician who performs this procedure is the person best able to interpret and to prescribe for this condition. Right heart catheterization involves lower risk factors and less discomfort than the better known angiogram or left heart catheterization, the type performed for coronary artery disease. To receive drug treatment for PAH before having a comprehensive diagnostic workup could be dangerous or make the condition worse for those at risk.

Although I have not had serious lung problems for seven years, a brief review my history of lung sensitivity might jog readers' memories and motivate them to review their pulmonary histories.

My maternal grandmother wheezed from asthma. For as long as I can remember, she used an atomizer with an opiate. My mother, father, and stepfather were indoor smokers, as were my grandparents. Tobacco was part of our home atmosphere. My mother's later life was plagued by emphysema.

At age four, after being boarded at a convent orphanage for a year, I became ill with double pneumonia. I recall looking up at the oxygen tent over my bed. My mother, who had been temporarily too sick herself to care for us, used to say I nearly died. After recovering, I was reunited with my mother and extended maternal family. My mother remarried when I was eight, and we moved to a little rural town. Hay fever and bronchitis arrived regularly with the seasonal changes.

At twelve I began to study French horn. I was a skinny frail kid. My parents worried, hoping my playing the horn would strengthen my lungs. Their fear of lung disease derived from my stepfather's brother dying young from tuberculosis. In my mid-teens, I was exposed to fiberglass when the family worked together insulating our attic ceiling. After this, my bronchial sensitivity seemed to worsen.

At age twenty, I went through a pack of cigarettes a day for two months during a brief employment as a secretary. Since inhaling was painful, I puffed on my menthol flavored cigarettes just to mark time as I waded through typing assignments. After leaving this job, I never smoked again.

My son always remarked on my frequent coughing and throat-clearing, which I attributed to post-nasal drip and allergies, not realizing digestive ills may have contributed. Ten years ago, the coughing turned into wheezing. For three months, I wheezed day and night. I went back to my internist several times to tell him the antibiotic wasn't working. The drug was making me sicker and the wheeze wasn't going away. He ordered a chest x-ray.

"One lung is folded over," he said. "I think you have walking pneumonia." He gave me another antibiotic. Still walking, I continued to wheeze. The next time I showed up at my internist's office, he referred me for allergy tests.

After an hour or more with patches of possible allergens stuck to the surface of my skin, the specialist told me I was seriously allergic to molds. I had hives and a wheezing reaction to penicillin in my twenties, but never thought of implications of external exposures to mold. The allergist asked how many books were in the house and advised me to get rid of those older than twenty years. He also warned me about very old and very new carpeting, ditto for upholstery. New fabrics are often treated with chemicals that can be lung irritants. He gave me prescriptions for a medication and inhaler. Since, at the time, I was wholly focused on finding natural causes and solutions, I postponed the recommended drug therapy.

Giving away my beloved old, and not so old, books was hard; these books I had carried from school to school, from parsonage to parsonage since seminary. After getting more than a hundred books out of the house improved my breathing, I was still wheezing. I began to suspect mold was coming up through the radiators of the antiquated heating system of our rented Victorian house. The allergist wrote a letter enabling us to terminate our lease.

After completing the recommended changes in my physical environment, I was still wheezing now and then. I began to consider my emotional environment, since over the previous year I had suffered several life-changing losses. There was plenty of stress mixed with the mold, and surely one's breathing can be affected by depression or anxiety. My recent retirement from the counseling center where I was employed for nearly ten years represented a significant loss, especially of long-time friends and colleagues I was used to seeing every day. Also, just as I was beginning to bond with my two young grandchildren, my son and family moved to the West Coast. This last was the more difficult.

Eventually, I came to acknowledge that the real reason for my early retirement was unresolved health issues, digestive and pulmonary. I had systemic scleroderma and didn't know it. The wheezing had greatly diminished, but not yet disappeared.

The summer after I left the counseling center, I went to Shalem (Hebrew word for "wholeness") Institute in Baltimore to begin seminars for a two-year program in spiritual direction. Classes met every day in a library holding volumes more than 1,000 years old. The resident monks were proud of their books. On the first day of the seminars, I began to wheeze so badly after the first couple of hours, I was ready to go home. A pastoral counselor in the group rescued me by offering the use of a little black box, which hung from a cord around his neck: a personal ionizer that ran on AA batteries. He explained how the ionizer clears the air around the face when there is pollution. I wore his ionizer around my neck for the rest of the week.

For this canary in the coal mine, the little black box kept me on my perch.

After a few days, other students in the seminar became sick with coughs and sinus problems. Later, in my investigation of the library space, I found mold in the window's air conditioning filter. On the days our seminar met outside, even with the bugs and the heat, breathing was reportedly easier for all affected.

After returning home, I purchased a personal ionizer advertised online. I wore the box around my neck when visiting parishioners in old houses. The ionizer I chose was able to remove eighty percent of smoke in the air around one's face. Old houses often harbor mold, especially in upholstery and carpeting that may have been absorbing moisture every rainy spring for half a century. Occasionally, a cigarette-smoking parishioner would apologize when he saw me switch on the little breathing machine. For me, the ionizer was effective against smoke, mold, and other common pollutants. Perfumes, scented candles, and room deodorizers still send me out the door.

Ultimately, I fled to South Florida in search of healing for my lung sensitivities. I recalled readings by Edgar Cayce prescribing the benefits of the seaside, particularly of sand. I imagined lying in hot dry sand closest to the surf and covering my chest with the weight of those tiny miraculous grains. I called a realtor friend and found an apartment on the East Coast at a reduced March rate. Since Bob also was retired, we embarked without hesitation. Every morning, for a month, I swam in the ocean before the noonday heat. I breathed salt air around the clock. I lay underneath the sand as I had dreamed. I relaxed. I waited. I prayed, asking for healing, and to find out what next I might do in my life.

While in Florida, I began to notice serious reflux after eating. Unaware of the dangers, including the possible relationship of this symptom to my lung issues, I resisted drug treatment. Fortunately, within a couple of weeks of beginning my self-prescribed sea-cure, the wheezing stopped.

Returning to New York State, Bob and I moved to a house we rented after obtaining permission to make specific repairs including a thorough cleaning of the heating system. We shouldered the expense of removing the decaying carpet, sanding the floors, and hiring professionals, first to flush out all the air ducts, and next to connect a complex filtering system to the gas furnace. Since then, I have remained obsessively careful about spaces I inhabit, even for a brief time.

Wednesday, June 4, 2008

Went to a reception for a parishioner soon to be married. Sat for two hours in the couple's charming, recently acquired old house and sank into a comfortable old couch. Either the wood beams or the upholstery were infected with mold, because I was coughing after the first hour; later on, a slight wheezing alarmed me.

A friend sitting on the couch with me whispered, "I'm allergic to something here; my eyes are tearing." We got out of there.

Saturday, June 14, 2008

Had to dress and fly to sing with a choir for the wedding. We practiced an hour in the loft and sang for another hour during the ceremony. The temperature in the sanctuary must have been 100 degrees. Coughing from a singer's hairspray, and in no shape for the reception, I made a beeline for the exit.

At home, answered some correspondence and emailed the choir director, excusing myself from singing for tomorrow's service as I'd promised. Self-protection's moving higher on my list of priorities.

Sunday, June 20, 2008

Staying at Nathalie's the last two nights after our trip to the Jersey shore. The central air conditioning in this house requires I wear a long-sleeved shirt and sweater. My nose is cold, my fingers, icy. Hope the air conditioning turns off automatically when the outdoor temperature rises. I'd like to open a window in my room.

Lots of old books, magazines, and antique furniture upstairs and down. In the living room a tapestry-covered chair sparked my suspicion for mold; it's awfully hard to breathe in there. Had an attack of coughing bordering on a wheeze before supper. Have to find way to get more comfortable here; I need to sleep.

Wednesday, July 23, 2008

This last night of the chaplains' retreat, everyone was invited to a party at the handicapped-accessible apartment of a participant. Most of us were staying in typical dorm rooms with no air conditioning and no space to spare. After a few minutes in the living room, I began to have trouble breathing. Mold in the carpet or in the upholstered furniture? Carol, who happens to have multiple sclerosis, also experienced asthma-like symptoms. After briefly lamenting the situation, we went out under the trees to continue our conversation, breathing fine.

Friday, July 25, 2008

Had pain in my right shoulder blade all day; it's worse when I take a deep breath. Remembering Wednesday night's coughing at the party, I want to make sure my lungs are okay. My chiropractor will check them later. Swimming partially relieved the ache, so it's probably muscular. I get scared when I have trouble breathing. Breathing is a big thing for people with SSc. Breathing is a big thing for everyone.

Tuesday, November 25, 2008

Coughing hard every time we practice in the church where we're performing this weekend. Drippy nose, too. Been taking an antihistamine before rehearsals. Could there be mold in that immense uncarpeted space? Could there be toxins jumping out from those 100-year-old wooden pews? Saturday morning I'll try not taking the antihistamine. The down side of the drug is a dry mouth and papery tongue. Not good for singers or speakers.

Wednesday, January 21, 2009

Met co-op neighbor in the hallway; she asked about my installation of the kitchen backsplash. When I told her about my conflict between choosing toxic tube glue or putting up with the smelly messiness of non-toxic contact cement, she suggested contact tape. Contact tape. Called Bob who said he'd pick up a roll on the way. In no time, we had the puzzle of perfectly cut embossed panels installed. And a thank-you note for under the door of my neighbor down the hall. Breathing easier.

SELF-CARE OPTIONS

Food and Medications

Protect against GERD through diet and prescribed medications. Stomach acid, when accidentally breathed into the lungs, can cause cumulative damage.

Indoor Air

Quality indoor air can be maintained as long as one's town or city has not been polluted by floods or recently targeted by other environmental disasters. Do not smoke or spend time in a house where others smoke. Avoid scented candles, air fresheners, potpourri, soaps, and strong cleaning agents, especially those containing chlorine or ammonia.

The most comprehensive approach to purifying indoor air is to have living and working space examined by professionals who can make an evaluation and informed recommendations. Heating and electrical systems, chemicals used in the building materials as well as those which may be in the soil under the house or building foundation are potential sources of indoor pollution. Most are remediable.

Wood and quality vinyl or marble floors are easier to keep allergen-free than carpeting. A newly installed carpet may require a person with lung sensitivity to wait weeks before using the space. A non-ionizing room air purifier with replaceable filters may be helpful.

Watch out for the things that may cause coughing or wheezing. Consider buying a personal ionizer for temporary use in spaces where smoke or mold may be present.

Household objects, including furniture, require careful inspection with respect to individual sensitivities. For instance, a dust allergy may exclude carpeted floors. An allergy to cat fur means no cat in the house unless one is willing to go for regular allergy injections. If feathers are on the verboten list, don't sleep on a down-filled pillow. Even newsprint can cause an allergic reaction in certain people. Read in a well-ventilated area; wash your hands, and discard.

In summary, we must continue to develop our awareness about what we can and cannot tolerate in the air we breathe.

Outdoor Air

We cannot, as individuals, control the quality of the outside air. Some people move to the Arizona desert for warm dry air; some move to Colorado for mountain air, and some, to warm coastal regions for ocean air. Most people, however, are unwilling or unable to move at all. Carry a filtering mask for self-protection from unexpected pollution when traveling. In the coldest weather, wear a mask or scarf that covers the mouth.

HEART

"I love you with all my heart and a little piece of my superior vena cava."

~A valentine from my son at age ten

Central to the circulatory system is the left ventricle of the heart which pumps oxygen-carrying blood, first through the aorta, then to a network of branching arteries, and ultimately to the tiny capillaries. We think, we move, we breathe, we heal in accordance with the ability of this system to carry sufficient oxygen from our head to our toes. Raynaud's Syndrome, which affects the fingers and sometimes the toes, is a case in point. When tiny blood vessels become narrowed, oxygen to these extremities may become extremely limited or cut off.

There are three ways disease mechanisms in SSc can affect the heart. When the heart muscle has scar tissue forming throughout, there is danger of *congestive heart failure* (CHF). This may be treated with steroids as, to date, there are no other reliably effective treatments.

Arrhythmias are abnormal heart rhythms, rhythms that are too fast, too slow, or irregular. These may be caused by scar tissue getting in the way of the electrical system that coordinates the beating of both sides of the heart muscle. Electrocardiogram and echocardiogram are the tests given to diagnose this condition. Depending upon the type of arrhythmia, medication or a pacemaker may be advised.

The third scleroderma-related heart illness is *pericarditis* caused by inflammation of the lining which surrounds the heart. The degree of seriousness depends upon whether or not the resulting accumulation of fluid pressing around the heart interferes with its ability to fill. This can be diagnosed by an echocardiogram. Although sometimes recurrent, pericarditis is a temporary condition responsive to steroid medications or to a surgical procedure, the purpose of which is to create a "window" that redirects the fluid buildup into the lung and is re-absorbed into the bloodstream.

Arteries and larger blood vessels also are subject to fibrosis, or hardening. In an illustrative diagram, this would present a picture similar to those that show clogging by cholesterol-generated plaque, or blood fat. In SSc, however, this vessel-narrowing is due to proliferation of collagen deposits. Artery walls thicken, and vessel linings can be slowly obliterated by this process. In the persons with systemic scleroderma, the damage to vessel walls and overproduction of collagen are the chief enemies of blood vessel function.

Before 1996, there were few effective treatments for pulmonary arterial hypertension (PAH). Many persons died from complications and organ failure. Oxygen, one of the early therapies, may still provide support; however, oxygen alone is insufficient over the long term. New inroads in pharmacological drugs are now keeping patients mobile and functioning for years. Most recently, organ transplantation has provided renewal of respiratory and heart function for a small number of critically ill persons.

About five years ago, I was diagnosed with an interatrial septal aneurysm. Whether this condition unrelated to SSc developed over years or was present at birth is unknown. The defect is represented by a weakened spot on the atrium wall, which can be monitored by a yearly echocardiogram and periodic "bubble tests." The condition presents no danger as long as the outgoing red blood and the incoming blue blood stay on their respective sides. If, however, a hole begins to form, there is a surgical procedure during which a reinforcing patch is sewn over the spot.

In my early thirties, I suffered what appeared to be an angina attack. I called in sick to the hospital where I was working as a counseling intern. Breathing was so painful; I stayed in bed for three days except for getting up to eat and go to the bathroom. After the pain subsided, I went back to work, never knowing the cause or diagnosis.

SELF-CARE OPTIONS
General Heart Care Tips

Scleroderma patients with or without mild heart abnormalities often require yearly echocardiograms.

Eat a variety of wholesome foods that are relatively low in saturated fats and high in antioxidants. With a doctor's approval, use a vitamin-E supplement and a teaspoon of omega-3, or flaxseed oil. B 12 and vitamin D are also important vitamins for heart health; recommended amounts vary with the individual.

Find the right exercise program. The type and intensity of exercise should be monitored by a physician and/or physical therapist.

Reduce negative stress wherever possible. Maintain loving relationships. Be intentional about caring for the interests of people closest to your heart and community, as well as for those at a distance who may be in greater need.

Sleep is critical to heart function. Persons who snore regularly, and/or experience periods of waking during the night, should to be checked for sleep apnea, as untreated sleep apnea can result in heart damage or stroke.

KIDNEYS

"I was born with music inside me. Music was one of my parts.
Like my ribs, my kidneys, my liver, my heart."
                    ~Ray Charles, American pianist, and singer, (1930-2004)

Our kidneys are made up of countless tiny blood vessels that weave in and around tube-like structures called nephrons, which assist in the removal of wastes from the blood. The cleansed blood flows back upward to the heart, while the separated wastes are excreted though the urine.

In persons who have SSc, blood vessels that supply the kidneys are prone to changes similar to those in the fingers or lungs. There are, in fact, medical references to "renal Raynaud's." Thickening of the vessel walls can interfere significantly with blood vessel flow, and, therefore, kidney function. The kidneys respond by releasing a hormone *renin,* which may cause a gradual or sudden potentially calamitous rise in blood pressure. This blood pressure rise in scleroderma is called *malignant hypertension,* and represents a renal crisis; this occurs in approximately twenty percent of the population with diffuse scleroderma. There are recognized risk factors. Patients with rapidly progressive skin-thickening on the truck and lower legs are more likely than others to be victims of this occurrence. Cardiac issues, anything that decreases cardiac output, may precipitate such an increase in blood pressure. Since there can be no completely reliable prediction about if, or when, malignant hypertension will strike, at-home blood pressure taking is recommended. Effective therapy exists; early intervention can be both kidney-saving and life-saving.

Also important is obtaining a clear diagnosis of PAH, a condition that has a way of hiding from the eyes of skilled specialists and is difficult to detect from a physical examination. Sometimes the patient needs to be proactive, not simply by asking the right questions, but by seeking out a pulmonary or cardiology specialist who can order and interpret tests appropriate to the symptoms.

Where there is any question of a vulnerability to malignant hypertension, the best investment may be the purchase of a quality blood pressure cuff. Your doctor can advise you about how often to check your pressure. Interpretation will depend on a comparison with normal pressure readings. Seek medical guidance about how to watch for and to respond to a gradual or sudden pressure rise.

Since the 1980s there have been major inroads to the treatment of malignant hypertension. ACE inhibitors (angiotensin-converting enzyme inhibitors) are central to managing and resolving these events. Early recognition is essential to a good outcome. With immediate therapy, kidney function can return to normal. When therapy is delayed, dialysis may be required; but with the use of ACE inhibitors, fifty percent of afflicted individuals recover sufficiently to come off dialysis.

At present, the manner in which SSc progresses or remits remains a mystery for the most part. In working toward a cure, we are each called to make our contributions to research and to raising awareness in whatever way we can.

SELF-CARE OPTIONS

Castor Oil Packs

Kidney health may be supported by applying castor oil packs to the back, over the location of these organs. This suggestion is my own and based entirely on the general healing properties of castor oil as evidenced in Edgar Cayce's work.

Food

There are prescribed diets for people on dialysis, with fluid restrictions. For persons without kidney issues a diet low in sugar and fat, and generous in fresh vegetables, whole grains, and fruits, generally will suffice. Pure water is always the best beverage. A popular drink suspected to harm kidney function, and sometimes vetoed by physicians, is dark cola because of its high potassium content. Cranberries and cranberry juice area believed to encourage kidney health.

Testing and Blood Pressure Monitoring

If a blood relation has diabetes, a yearly hemoglobin A1C blood test may be a wise precaution. This test shows the average blood sugar level for the previous three months. Quite independently from a diagnosis of SSc, kidney health may be in jeopardy when blood sugar levels remain high.

For scleroderma patients who have risk factors for malignant hypertension, home blood pressure monitoring is essential. Failure to recognize a sudden rise in blood pressure can result in temporary or permanent kidney damage. Consult your doctor about when and how to proceed.

PART II
THE MEDICAL/SELF-CARE INTERFACE

Chapter 5
TESTS AND PROCEDURES

"Learned helplessness is the giving-up reaction, the quitting response
that follows from the belief that whatever you do doesn't matter."
~Arnold Schwarzenegger

Most people with scleroderma require regular tests, screenings, and procedures essential for identifying changes in the function and/or chemistry of the body's systems. The patient may experience himself/herself being pricked, prodded, chilled, and cruelly invaded on a regular basis. Although we may seldom complain, medical tests, particularly, invasive procedures may encourage a sense of helplessness. Laboratory and treatment rooms can become places where we feel victimized, especially during periods when we are most vulnerable.

"What are they going to do to me?" is a question seldom asked aloud. At best, we will determine to put off such thoughts. At worst, we will tough it out. Many people are timid about speaking up in medical settings. There's an inner prompter: "Say yes; be nice. Don't bother anyone. If you do, they could get mad and hurt you more."

At my internist's, I was asked: "Okay for the nurse trainee to give you the shot?"

"Sure," I answered, and then, "Ouch!"

The trainee, clearly nervous, had flubbed the injection. She prepared to try again. Would it be "Ouch!" again? Taking courage to intervene on my own behalf, I asked for someone else to administer the shot.

Making notes about one's experience both before and after tests and procedures may be helpful in managing and negotiating future testing situations. Writing externalizes internal monologue and can generate ideas about how better to prepare for the next scheduled round.

Because there are a vast number of diagnostic tests, procedures, and screenings across the medical spectrum, this summary will be limited to those I have undergone. Over the past several years, I have tried to bring creative preparation, negotiation, and follow-up into various testing situations to minimize discomfort and to maximize a sense of control over my experience in laboratories and treatment rooms.

Learning to ask for blankets or information when in a laboratory setting can set the stage not only for a more relaxed experience but, in some instances, for test results that are closer to a true reading of one's present condition.

Blood Work

Whether trips for blood work are monthly or biannually, whether they are after a night of fasting or after lunch, there are ways to change this experience from being one more stressor to a brief interruption in the day.

The turning point for me was early one morning when I noticed a tremor in the hands of my assigned phlebotomist. While searching for a vein, he stabbed me more than once. Because of his tremor, the needle jiggled when he changed vials. Although I endured in silence, this blood draw motivated me to act in the selection of my phlebotomists.

> Thursday, May 22, 2008
>
> Spoke up at the lab this morning. The nurse at the window suggested a phlebotomist who is good with the butterfly needle, but warned that I'd have to wait longer than if I took my turn with the lab person more immediately available. Hardly opened my book before being called by a virtuoso phlebotomist whose "pinch" was really a pinch. Her first name and work schedule are recorded in my appointment book for easy access.

Colonoscopy

Because persons with SSc and other autoimmune diseases are prone to intestinal problems, this procedure may be performed more often on them than on those in the general population.

To facilitate entry and visibility, the colon is expanded with air. A tiny camera and surgical instruments are guided upward through the lower bowel; the walls of the colon are shown on a computer monitor. Visual examination may indicate the need for particular attention onsite during the procedure, which usually lasts about half an hour.

In my third-year follow-up of a colonoscopy with polyps removal, my GI specialist suggested a new preparation prescription, a simple pill to be taken after supper on the night before the procedure. I asked, instead, to be given the familiar prep, the one that includes a day-long liquid fast with the voluminous nasty drink. My reason for the choice: I had heard that some physicians believe the old preparation provides better visibility of the colon walls.

I dreaded becoming physically weak during and after the liquid fast. In the past, I would get a bad headache and feel faint. The prescribed liquid diet includes clear bullion, light-colored juices, flavored gelatins, and popsicles. These foods translate to salt, water, and sugar, with some vitamin content in the juice, and some protein in the prepared gelatin dessert. Intended to satisfy the specialist's requirement for a clean colon, these foods also may be intended to encourage patient compliance, as they require little or no preparation.

I have developed, what is for me, an optimal liquid fast. A touch of apple juice in drinking water may support alkalinity of the GI tract. Powdered unsweetened gelatin can be warmed and added to the apple juice for a tasty protein without extra sugar. I simmered fresh chicken parts in a package of organic chicken broth, and shoulder lamb chops in another, removing meat and parsley after cooking. The homemade meat broths must be refrigerated in order to harden the fat for removal. Also, they must be reheated and strained to qualify as "clear bullion." Although work and time intensive, the payoff for me was feeling stronger both before and after a colonoscopy.

You might consider packing your own food and drink for breaking the fast in the recovery area. If you bring your own, make a list to show the admitting nurse on the day of your procedure. Opening unreported containers in the recovery area might cause suspicion. Some hospitals serve soup and a sandwich if you are there around lunchtime. The hospital I have used for GI procedures offers a muffin with coffee or soda for breakfast, alien fare for a gluten-free, caffeine-free individual.

When I requested light sedation for a recent colonoscopy, my GI doctor said some people have the procedure with zero sedation, suggesting I might be interested in remaining conscious for the adventure. Doubtful, but curious, I held off with the anesthetic until shortly after the procedure had begun. Uncomfortable cramping led to my asking for a little anesthesia, after which I was lost for the duration.

DEXA, Bone Scan

Having SSc may set one up for decreased bone density. There are theories that point to the influence of certain vitamins, medications and foods that may lead either to an increase or decrease in bone density. As long as bone density falls within the normal range for one's age, bone scans every two years are advised. However, when osteopenia or osteoporosis is present, a doctor may write an order to repeat the DEXA after a single year to test the effectiveness of specific therapies, including drugs that have been prescribed.

A DEXA or bone scan is an easy test to take. While wearing the loose scrubs provided, one lies briefly on a table, which in my experience has never felt particularly cold.

Echocardiogram

The echocardiogram, an ultrasound test for viewing and recording heart function, may also reveal pulmonary hypertension. In SSc, a change in size and/or function of the right and left chambers, or atriums, can be indicators of fibrosis or hardening of blood vessels, arteries, and even the heart muscle itself.

Although one must remove all clothes from above the waist, the only discomfort during this exam may be the body's first contact with the moisturizing cream for enabling smooth movement of the radiological instrument over the skin. If the rest of one's body is warm, this should not be a problem. In cool treatment rooms, I have asked for towels to cover shoulders and portions of my chest not being immediately scanned.

Eye Tests

Persons with systemic scleroderma have increased susceptibility to normal-tension, also called low-tension, glaucoma. This condition is believed to be caused by an inherited fragility of the optic nerve, or the result of blocked blood flow through the tiny capillaries that supply it. A visual field, optic nerve photo, and optical coherence tomography (OCT), which is a laser scan of the optic nerve fibers, may all be used in confirming diagnosis. Since, with low-tension glaucoma, intraocular pressure may vary within in the normal range, pressure checks alone are inconclusive.

Open-angle glaucoma, also often inherited, is a common treatable condition. I received this diagnosis twenty years ago. I have three tests on a regular basis: tomography, or pressure check; visual field tests; and optic nerve photos. None of these is particularly uncomfortable. The photo test creates an after-shock from the bright lights shined directly into the eyes; I need fifteen minutes to a half hour before reading or driving. The OCT laser scan, with which I have no experience, also is performed with light.

Although eye drops can sting, cause redness and more disturbing side effects, my therapy for open-angle glaucoma remained comfortably stable for years.

Those with SSc are more likely than the general population to have a dry-eye condition. An ophthalmologist can be helpful with this and offer many options. I treat this with chemical-free eye drops, a mineral oil application, and other at-home therapies to keep the lashes clean, and eyes and lids warm and well hydrated. There is a new drug on the market as well as a laser procedure called SLT, or selective laser trabeculoplasty, which are used to lower optic pressure and increase tear production. The new laser treatment does not produce scarring.

Gastrointestinal Endoscopies

The upper endoscope procedure involves the GI specialist viewing the esophagus all the way from its opening in the throat to the stomach. Portions of the stomach as well as the entire esophagus are visible by way of a miniscule camera. The camera, along with other tiny instruments, is swallowed by the lightly anesthetized patient. This procedure ought to be painless with no painful aftermath unless excessive surgical intervention is required.

Friday, February 27 2009

Emailed my Albany rheumatologist about whether I'm neurotic to be wondering whether I really need to have the endoscope procedure right away. Since stopping my calcium capsules, eating has been easier. Guess I'd like to be certain swallowing the miniature camera, scraper, and dilator is really necessary to my health.

Sunday, March 1, 2009

In my fragile understanding of this life, I often stand in the crosswinds of science and faith. If I listen to my inner voice about the upcoming procedure, the solution is simple; all I need to do is watch my sleep. If I sleep well again tonight, I'll be fine about going ahead with the procedure. If I sleep poorly, I'll be tempted to cancel and confer with the GI doctor later on. Is that crazy? Don't think so. Intuition has nearly always worked better for me than raw logic.

Monday, March 2, 2009

Albany rheumatologist's email response came today. He wrote: "Questioning an upcoming procedure is a natural part of the process leading to a decision."

My decision already is one of acceptance. There is definitely something wrong at the esophageal junction. Grateful for another sound sleep, I'm becoming almost eager about Wednesday's procedure. Last night a singer from The Madrigal Choir who teaches nursing helped confirm my observation that an upper endoscope procedure is much simpler than a colonoscopy. By looking at an anatomical diagram, anyone can see the straight path from gullet to gut. She knows my GI specialist and reassured me he will honor my request to go light on the sedation.

Wednesday, March 4, 2009

This is the day. As soon as I lay on the treatment table, I felt cold: the air conditioning. Put my hands under my thighs, trying to snuggle under the thin sheet, which I pulled up to my chin. Clueless about hospital hygiene, Bob offered to cover me with my down-filled coat. I screwed up my courage to ask the nurse for a warm blanket and was soon relaxed under a microwaved flannel cover.

The nurse came to attach the oximeter to my fingertip for measuring oxygen saturation.

"It's not warm enough yet," I told her, holding up a purple-tipped index finger, a victim of Raynaud's: "My ear would work better."

She put the oximeter on my finger anyway.

Getting me connected to the IV also failed on the first try. All the veins in my hand and forearm had suddenly vanished. She tried another angle, but no blood would flow through the tubing. Removing the IV catheter hurt more than its installation. I was stoic.

Success on the second try. She found at the top of my right hand a cooperative vein sticking out a little more than the others.

Having sucked all the warmth out of the heated blanket, I was mustering the courage to ask for a second, hoping they'd wheel me out and sedate me before I got too cold. I'd rather interrupt an aide than a nurse, but can't tell one from the other when they are all wearing those cheery bunny-bear shirts over white slacks. I called to the nearest bunny-bear-shirted woman in the hallway. Warm again under two heated blankets, I had only to remember to make my preoperative declaration before slipping away: verification of my name and birth date, and a reminder to the doctor that I have scleroderma and, finally, ask him to go light on the sedation.

I saw my oxygen saturation increase dramatically on the monitor screen immediately after the oximeter was taken off my cold index finger and clipped to my hot ear. All was well. Closed my eyes and sank into the soft darkness.

Coming to and wondering what mad things I may have uttered while under the influence, I asked the attending nurse if I had been helpful during the procedure. She said "yes."

During a past endoscopy, there were directives about swallowing and counting backwards, and some pain and singing, yes, singing before I relinquished consciousness. I still have a little trepidation about authority figures, even those wearing bunny-bear shirts.

Thursday, March 26, 2009

After a good sleep, enjoyed a day of work and rest in the right proportions; began to rearrange client hours for next week, fixing my schedule to accommodate Friday morning's procedure. This will be my second upper endoscopy in five weeks. The purpose is to see if, or how much, the ulcer has healed and to take tissue from underneath the ulcer site for biopsy.

Friday 3, April 2009

Today was all about getting the procedure over with and finding out what's what. Much easier this time, asking for those microwaved blankets. A workable vein for the IV was immediately found. Waking in the treatment room to hear the doctor say that the ulcer was 100 percent healed, followed by overwhelming gratitude.

Except for sharing a small soup meal with Bob, I slept rest of the day, mostly from relief. During the later hours, I slept more from a need to hide from the world as long as possible.

Under some circumstances the patient or patient's advocate may need to initiate inquiry about diagnostic testing. If the patient is unable to communicate with medical staff, a family member or trusted friend may be appointed as advocate: someone with knowledge of the patient's disturbing new or unresolved symptoms. A person may be legally designated in advance to speak with the specialist or primary physician.

Essentially, I referred myself for the endoscopy procedure, which marked the beginning of my healing.

For patients who have mysterious symptoms from mysterious diseases, there is often no clear path to relief. To me, the frustration and suffering from more serious symptoms of systemic illnesses is hardly imaginable. Testing that can clarify the medical picture and point toward helpful therapies needs to be made available, as well as reasonably pain-free, whenever possible.

Mammograms, Breast Biopsies, Pap Tests

I was surprised to learn that persons with systemic scleroderma and other autoimmune diseases are more likely to get cancer than other people. While yearly mammograms are advised for all women, they are especially important for the older population since the statistical possibility of cancer increases with age. The new digital radiological instruments are able to detect micro-calcifications which, in eighty percent of cases, indicate benign or non-cancerous cells. The possibility of falling into the twenty percent of malignant findings is a reminder that one's yearly mammogram could be life-saving.

There are ways of remaining as relaxed as possible during a mammogram or biopsy, although the latter naturally elicits more concern. These are: stay warm, be sufficiently nourished, and maintain a positive cooperative, if not meditative, attitude. If you tend to get cold in air-conditioned treatment rooms, ask the nurse or attendant who gave you the thin cotton robe to bring you a second or heavier robe or a blanket.

With needle or core biopsy procedures, surgeon, nurse, and radiologist may all be present in the treatment room. There is light compression of the breast, administration of a local anesthetic, and in my case there was little or no subsequent pain. A re-freezable soft pad may be offered for applying at intervals during the first days. Every effort may be made to support and relax the patient, including explaining the procedure step by step. In the event explanations are not forthcoming, the patient can request them in the moment.

Key to having a painless Pap smear is intentional relaxation. Deep breaths and trust have usually worked for me.

In the waiting area, there may be a selection of beverages, fresh fruit, and cookies. If you think you will require more solid nutrition, pack up before you go. More nutritious food may be brought from home. When waiting in cool treatment areas which threaten to bring on a Raynaud's attack, I have worn gloves or mittens. My favorites have a removable cap over the tops of the fingers which enable page-turning. Wearing gloves into an X-ray or treatment room may prompt questions from the nurse or technician, which is an opportunity to raise their awareness about Raynaud's.

Clinicians in gynecological and breast care centers are well aware of patients' anxiety when undergoing these procedures, but they may have little awareness of SSc symptoms and the dangers inherent in overlooking them.

> Sunday, May 10, 2009
>
> Went in for mammogram and Pap smear, was seen by the nurse practitioner who examined my breasts and took the smear while we talked amicably about nutrition, exercise, and how differently women age. Both were easy because I was relaxed and warm.

Pulmonary Function Test

This test is ordered regularly for scleroderma patients who have suspected non-progressive fibrosis, slight hardening of lung tissue, which may impair lung strength and capacity. The test takes about one hour and can be tiring.

People with claustrophobia may become extremely uncomfortable sitting in the chair enclosure, a formidable challenge even for the non-claustrophobic. Fortunately, the walls of the plethysmography box, commonly referred to as "the body box," are made of glass so the patient can see through them. The respiratory therapist who administers the test stands reassuringly near. She may offer helpful coaching, which enables the patient to attain the best possible score by making several practice tries.

During the last part of the test, the door to the glass chamber is firmly closed. At this point a number of people reportedly experience intense anxiety, even panic. The most effortful part of the test occurs now, with the pushing the air from one's lungs against a measurement barrier.

Several years ago while undergoing my first, or baseline, pulmonary function test, by which future PFTs are measured; I had trouble getting an airtight seal of my lips over the mouthpiece. My dental bridge appliance appeared to be the problem. Even when I removed the appliance, loss of elasticity in the muscles around my mouth made this adaptation quite a struggle. I wanted to achieve the most accurate reading so I would not appear to have less lung volume than I actually had.

The respiratory therapist patiently assisted me during an hour of surprisingly hard work. She said, for persons with a narrowed mouth or decreased oral aperture, a pediatric mouthpiece is available and usually solves the problem of getting an airtight seal. The therapist suggested a technique helpful to me, but one which may prove difficult or impossible for persons with severe hand or finger impairment. She showed me how to hold my hands against my cheeks close to the corners of my mouth to get an airtight seal when blowing into the measuring device.

Over several years, I have become more confident in taking the pulmonary function test, which may have contributed to the improved results.

Six-Minute Walk Test

This test measures the oxygen saturation level as the patient walks at a brisk pace alongside the respiratory therapist. The measuring device is usually attached to the index finger which can be a poor conductor if one has Raynaud's.

> Thursday, April 16, 2009
>
> Spent most of the afternoon at the hospital. For the first time, the six-minute walk test was enjoyable. Usually, I'm walked like Spot, the dog, around hospital corridors, my leash, the cord connecting my oximeter finger to the respiratory therapist's palm-sized computer. I must have been a strange

sight, swinging my arms back and forth, Frankenstein-style, to get oxygen down into my fingertips. Today I caught a glimpse out the windows of spring blues and greens. The indoor scenery is hospital wall art. I impulsively suggested we go outdoors.

To my surprise, the respiratory therapist led me out of the building, and we walked in the sunshine. The spring air was warm. Grass, trees, and flowers surrounded us. We walked around the perimeter of a hospital building, careful to fulfill requirements for time and pacing. Keep in mind that not all respiratory therapists are free to take the outdoor walk.

Chapter 6
PHYSICIANS AND OTHER PRACTITIONERS

"Everyone has a doctor in him or her. We just have to help it in its work."
~Hippocrates, Greek Physician, 460-377 B.C.

The most important physician in the healing network of most people with systemic scleroderma is the rheumatologist. Like others in our region's Scleroderma Foundation support group, I consult with two rheumatologists. If you live in or near a small city, there are advantages of having a trusted specialist nearby, in addition to having a specialist who practices in a larger city. My local rheumatologist who was instrumental in my diagnosis is involved in coordinating my care, and available to respond to scleroderma-related health issues without my having to drive long distances for consultations. A scleroderma specialist is more likely to be involved in clinical research and probably has treated a larger number of patients with SSc than small city doctors, and may offer a different slant on alternative choices.

I am fortunate to have a trusting relationship with both rheumatologists. Each is highly credentialed and has worked in group practice for many years. My local specialist and I have sung in The Madrigal Choir for more than a decade. I was referred to my Albany specialist by a mutual friend, also a physician, and member of the Choir.

Other doctors who are part of my healing network are an internist, a gastrointestinal specialist, and an ophthalmologist. I see a cardiologist every few years. As yet, I have no pulmonary specialist.

My ancillary practitioners are or have been: a chiropractor, a naturopathic doctor, a therapeutic massage therapist, a podiatrist, a dentist; and, most recently, a physical therapist. My experiences of working with each of these individuals, specialists in their own right, may be found in this section, as well as throughout the journal notes.

Sometimes I have joked about how I try to choose my "witch doctors" as carefully as I choose traditional doctors. Practitioners of traditional medicine may utilize modalities from both tested and speculative resources. Individuals who operate outside the boundaries of the Federal Drug Association (FDA) and the National Institute of Healing (NIH) include some highly respected physicians.

At the risk of being considered irrational by those empirically and/or scientifically minded, I include two practitioners in my healing network, both of whom walked the earth before our time. They are Edgar Cayce and Jesus of Nazareth. Neither ascribed medical skills or training to themselves, nor had any. Jesus, who has been called "The Great Physician," I credit with influencing a long line of women and men whose greatness, whatever their skills and training, is revealed through greatness of spirit. Jesus, from the Heavenly Realm, brought presence, prayer, word, and touch. Cayce, a follower of Jesus, revealed a deeply contemplative spirit, using prayer and natural foods as well as applications of castor bean and nutritive oils in his healing work. Cayce also prescribed the use of a wet cell appliance for his scleroderma patients, an apparatus I have never seen, but would like to investigate.

Although Edgar Cayce had little general education and no medical training, he helped thousands of seriously ill people return to health. He was balanced and low-key in his manner. While in an altered state or trance with his wife and secretary taking notes, Cayce diagnosed and prescribed for each patient. Although his non-traditional methods have kept many from taking his work seriously, I regard him as a true representative of systematic contemplative discipline, and a practitioner whom I continue to admire and meditatively consult.

Documentation of over 9,000 of Cayce's readings are kept in files and distributed by the Association for Research and Enlightenment (A.R.E.) in Virginia Beach, Va. In addition to his original notes, there are many books written about Cayce's work. In the 1980s I made a weekend pilgrimage to the A.R.E. library with an educator from my parish to read and attend workshops.

As long as we care for our own bodies as best we can and inquire in the right places, we may always have hope of healing. Hope is not a guarantee, and there are few research grants devoted to the study of lifestyle changes. An encouraging word from our physicians and other practitioners has the power to lift our spirits and, often, that is enough to give us the courage to carry on.

Doctors involved with their busy practices may not always consider the broad healing network that exists outside their treatment specialties. Rheumatologists routinely treat the symptoms of SSc, and at times must feel helpless in witnessing how this and related diseases wreck havoc on digestive, cardio-vascular, musculoskeletal, and other bodily systems.

We need to learn about and to watch for changes in our bodies, and be free to ask for a referral in dealing, alternatively, with a persistent pain or new finding. Every physician has the option, and sometimes the responsibility, to refer to another practitioner. When patients are willing and able to work more intensely on their health issues, referrals to counselors, physical and massage therapists, nutritionists, as well as to other healthcare professionals may encourage a patient's commitment to lifestyle changes, and lead to significant improvements in both attitude and function.

During intervals of greater health or remission, consultations and treatment by auxiliary practitioners may decrease. For some, there may be an ebb and flow in treatment by chiropractic, naturopathic, and massage therapists, especially when patients' balance within their body systems increases.

Wednesday, June 18, 2008

Good focused visit with my internist. Stuck to my fifteen minutes of questions and answers, got my next order for blood work including sedimentation rate which I've been curious about. Sedimentation rate involves measuring how long it takes for the red blood cells to sink into the drawn blood, and figures into an alternative treatment of SSc, a treatment with antibiotic therapy, developed by Thomas McPherson Brown, M.D. The work of the late Dr. Brown is supported by the Road Back Foundation. I toyed for a while with the idea of seeking this treatment.

Re: osteoporosis. My internist said keeping my vitamin-D level up may be as important as weight-bearing exercise. Although I can't believe an increase in any vitamin can win the battle, I'm going along with his recommendation to increase the amount of D, and continuing to have my blood levels monitored. As I was getting ready to leave, my doctor took out a new ACE bandage and wrapped my right wrist where I have an enlarged, sometimes painful, calcified bone. This immediately relieved the ache. I stopped him when he began to tell me about his children, certain he was late for his next patient. The new oversized clock on his office wall does not seem to have increased his awareness of time.

Friday, July 25, 2008

Chiropractor pronounced my shoulder pain muscular, probably from the icy air conditioning in the lecture room this week. He listened from every angle with the stethoscope, said my lungs are clear. Maybe I'm too careful, too quick to seek diagnostic interpretation. Yet I know with autoimmune diseases problems can emerge with little warning. Rare diseases involve rare sensitivities; I want to be ready to respond as early as possible to any change in my health picture.

Sunday, August 24, 2008

To be able to reach a medical practitioner on a Friday night is almost unheard of. My chiropractor was not only willing to take the time to help me through the most evil hour of reflux ever, but invited me to call back with a follow-up report on Saturday morning. He's been helping me through a hard year, but I need answers now neither he nor my physicians have been able to give me.

Friday, December 26, 2008

A friend who's the wife of a physician in town called to tell me about yesterday morning when her husband said he'd like to spend the day with "his cousin." Since neither of them has a living cousin, she asked who this might be.

"My cousin, Jesus," he said, referring with his quiet humor to his Jewish identity. So Christmas morning, the two served dinner to neighborhood people downtown, while I, a minister of the Gospel, was stuffing myself at two family feasts. I'm impressed how they went out of their way to serve a meal to strangers. His wife has the stress of a caretaking profession, also. I hope he saw his cousin in the people with nowhere else to go.

Physicians seem to have greater privacy and time considerations than the rest of us. I know, in a lesser way, from my own work, the difficulty of trying to keep the balance between self-care and caring for others. Wanting to do good to others can lure us into overdoing when confronted with human need. This becomes an awareness issue for anyone who takes on such a role or responsibility, from parent to physician, from teacher to counselor, from farmer to pastor.

Wednesday, January 28, 2009

The expensive shoes I ordered through the orthotic expert a month ago still are poking into my bunion and come off my heels when I walk. I've called and written to the expert; he hasn't answered. I think he's given up on me. I think I've given up on him.

Today I soaked my three-year-old canoe-shaped sandals in hot water and dried them in a warm oven to tighten the sides. For the past several years, this has been the only style I can wear with my bulky inserts for an entire day.

Saturday, February 7, 2009

Until I find a solution to this esophageal issue, I'm leaning heavily on Edgar Cayce's remedies: The castor oil pack on my chest, vegetable soup in a bowl, the "beef juice" broth being rendered in a pot on my stove. I'm doing everything I to help get past this low point.

Wednesday, February 11, 2009

The therapeutic massage therapist met me this afternoon in my office to discuss our bartering arrangement. A few weeks ago, while she was loosening my back muscles in the chiropractor's office, I asked if she might know a licensed massage therapist who'd be interested in exchanging an hour of massage for an hour of spiritual direction.

"I would," she answered without hesitation.

The idea began in my mind as an experiment, an intentional role reversal. If we follow up on our proposed arrangement, there's a possibility each of us might have some fears about disclosure. My client needs to feel trust before confiding details about her inner life, especially her spiritual life. Likewise, the massage therapist's client must experience a level of trust.

I'm worried I might lose credibility as a professional by lying almost naked on the massage table to be treated by a prospective "client." She has seen my curved spine in the chiropractor's office. I may be uncomfortable revealing other well-concealed imperfections. The ropey varicosities in my legs are evident even when I'm lying down; they show through the skin of my feet like tangled blue cords.

In my office I'm relatively confident of my appearance. A good haircut, a little make-up, coordinated slacks and jackets, render crookedness of spine and vein invisible. As for my unlovely feet, they're nearly always concealed by compression hose, which I must wear even in summer.

Saturday, February 21, 2009

In spite of my narcissistic concerns, I showed up for my first massage at 1:00 p.m. The treatment room is pleasant with muted lighting, though a bit chilly. From a CD in the corner came the voice of a woman singing. The therapist covered me with blankets and placed a heat pack on my back that, after a few moments, felt scalding.

I asked first for more insulation from the heat, and would she please replace the singing with instrumental music. A moment before I wondered: "As the designated client, can I ask for what I want when there is no money in the exchange?"

"This is your time," she said, agreeably; and provided a buffer for the heat pack and switched the CD to flutes. I can relax in the company of flutes.

There was a thoughtful, almost prayerful quality in her touch. Her fingers found the spaces between the connective tissue along my spine, tiny places, unused to motion. She moved them. We conversed easily from time to time; though, most of the hour, I basked in long silences, giving in to the enjoyment of my newly pliable self. The persistent winter ache in my right shoulder began to disappear.

Am surprised at how easily I was able to let my body be touched and loosened by someone who's scheduled to sit in my office next Wednesday. Surprised at myself, how lying almost naked on the massage table, I was able so quickly to relinquish concerns about bodily imperfections. After the massage, I dressed quickly and looked the in mirror to see the remarkable renewal, signs of age and wear melted away.

In the past I have enlisted massage therapists only to relieve a specific ache or pain. From my late thirties, every winter I sought massage to melt stiffness in my left shoulder. During my forties and fifties, I sought massage as well as chiropractic to ease a backache bad enough to keep me from getting in and out of my car. Most backaches seemed to come from sitting for too many hours in even the most comfortable office chair. This Saturday, though, I lay on the table not for the purpose of eliminating a specific pain. I hoped I might begin to understand how this form of hands-on treatment might promote general healing in a body that has grown used to a background of mild pain.

This experiment has started me thinking about the meaning of providing and receiving treatment. To be the practitioner means to accept one's self as caretaker for the duration of the treatment interval, to be the one who is willing and able to engage both the person and the disease, to say the healing word, to manipulate, to bind or soothe, and, at last, to offer helpful recommendations and/or a prescription. All these ministrations must be carried out with genuine humility so as not to risk shaming the patient. Because of having to disclose details of his or her "ugly wounds," those visible or invisible imperfections, the patient is more vulnerable to feeling shame.

Monday, March 2, 2009

My internist and I spoke on the phone about my upcoming endoscope procedure. He suggested I remind the GI doctor about my scleroderma, so he will note the possibility my tissue may be tighter and harder to stretch than the tissue of someone without a connective tissue disease. Never hesitate to remind doctors about specific concerns, particularly before invasive procedures, he said.

Saturday, March 28, 2009

The massage therapist discovered hidden muscle tightness, which she freed with skill and patience during my late afternoon treatment. She explained how just touching a sore spot on one's body can ease the hurt and sometimes eliminate the pain. Later in the hour, she also demonstrated foot reflexology by pulling on my toes one by one, and pressing the area on either side of each toe with thumb and forefinger. She showed me how I could do this myself.

We kiss our children's bruised knees; we rub their backs. How many of us think to carry out the simplest actions to relax and heal our own bodies?

Wednesday, April 15, 2009

Going for my massage was the joy of the week. First time ever I was able to lie face down on the treatment table without an attack of GERD. Hooray for my healed ulcer! I was lying on my back when she told me about the rectangular space on the upper chest, directly under my neck, bounded on each side by my shoulders.

"It's called 'the cloud gates,'" she said, "the seat of a person's creativity, the locus of poetry, music, art...."

"Perhaps even the healing arts," I added, as if science could bear the thought.

Chapter 7
GROUPS

"Redemption is the recognition that we are all part of the same family."
~Rabbi Lance J. Sussman, PhD
Temple Keneseth Israel, Elkins Park, PA

Many people stay closer to home after being diagnosed with a rare and unpredictable disease because they feel safer in familiar places. Two years passed before I found the courage to attend our regional support group, sponsored by the Scleroderma Foundation. A born introvert, most of my life I've had to practice being comfortable in rooms full of people. I understand well the longing to be quiet, to hunker down under the covers with a book, and to cancel a lunch date in the middle of January.

Serving congregations for nearly thirty years forced me to let go much of my self-protective shyness. I learned to welcome strangers, to take unfamiliar hands in mine in hospitals and funeral homes. I held parishioners and sometimes strangers in my arms at tragic junctures in their lives.

Moving outward into the world can benefit almost everyone. Whatever one's living arrangements, scheduled breaks from home and work settings are almost a necessity. Relationships between persons who live in the same household can be enriched by sharing interests outside their home. When accompanied by a Scleroderma Foundation member, single adults, friends, and whole family units are welcome at support group meetings.

There are many other worthwhile group options to consider as well, from community choral or orchestral groups to college classes. For me, singing and learning new skills have been an ongoing pleasure.

While the Internet provides a virtual way of reaching out to others, there is no substitute for real-life interaction. Some medical websites offer genuinely helpful information. Unfortunately, there is also Internet information that is misleading and may offer dangerous advice. Every meaningful human relationship goes beyond the exchange of information.

Because my son and family are a day's flight away, and other relatives more than a hundred miles distant, I have developed close friendships close to home. The friends I see most often have a firsthand understanding of my physical challenges, and I, of theirs. My relatives have only a sketchy idea gleaned from telephone conversations and infrequent visits. Although I can count on my family's good will and their love and prayers over the miles, our ability to appreciate one another's daily lives, including our respective health issues, is limited.

The people whom I see regularly, including Bob's family, which has become mine, the pastoral counseling staff, members of my swim, musical, exercise, support, and faith groups, my co-op neighbors, are the people who have expanded my concept of a healing network far beyond anything I could imagine.

Sunday, May 11 2008

Mother's Day's service went well. My son called from far away. Hearing my grandson's clear child voice saying "Happy Mother's Day" was a high point. Being in tune with the people in the congregation, with my family, with life, is a good place to be.

Sunday, May 19, 2008

During our Welsh concert, the audience joined The Madrigal Choir in singing many of the hymns. A few of the hymns we sang in Welsh. The Choir had been coached to articulate phonetically learned phrases, while a number of people in the pews knew the language well. Together we were a great harmonious mix of voices and perspectives.

Afterwards, friends Max and Geri came by for supper. We laughed and told stories in the way of old friends.

Thursday, June 5, 2008

Went solo to my first Scleroderma Foundation support group meeting tonight. Excitement mixed with anxiety. We met at a hospital near my co-op. A few members drive some distance to get there. Salads, fruit, and breads were arranged buffet-style on a long table. Several of the women brought husbands or boyfriends. We took turns introducing ourselves. Individuals' health issues spanned the continuum from temporary wellness to significant distress.

One man spoke of trust in his doctor, whom he travels hundreds of miles to see. I asked if his doctor is a rheumatologist.

"No," he replied, laughing. He's not just a rheumatologist; he is 'God!'" There was knowing laughter because several members of the group consult with the same specialist about whom the most striking fact is his scheduling of each new scleroderma patient for a three-hour consultation. Those caught in the maelstrom of this mysterious illness value time with our rheumatologists more than gold.

The focus on disease issues was secondary to the pleasure of being with people who are bright and unobtrusively friendly. The executive director's relaxed leadership style made my first meeting easier. At the close, she read a summary of the Tri-State Chapter's core mission statement printed on the handout:

"To provide educational and emotional support to people with scleroderma and their families. To stimulate and support research designed to identify the cause of scleroderma as well as improve methods of treatments. To enhance the public's awareness of this disease."

Friday, June 13, 2008

Mainline churches, with all their limitations, have been and continue to be places of healing for me. I serve several denominations as well as my own and experience every sanctuary as a hallowed place whether I'm guest preacher or visitor. I've felt a sense of belonging in the reform synagogue singing for the High Holy Days. Dedication to prayer and service invite a sacred energy we call the Holy Spirit, which blows where it will, and can turn strangers into friends.

Monday, July 14, 2008

Today was my mother's birthday. Do most people pause at the birth and death dates of their parents? Whenever I hear a solo violin, I remember how beautifully she played. Memories of family who have gone on are so much more real than the fading black-and-white photographs on top of my piano. Every day I set the table with the same English china we used in our row house when I was small and four generations of the maternal side lived together.

This morning I swam with the nine o'clock group. Weaving in and out of seven bobbing bodies, there's no room to swim laps, but I enjoy the camaraderie. Drying off in the sauna, I absent-mindedly rubbed my skin with shampoo instead of olive oil; both containers are the same size and shape. Broke everybody up when I had to get back into the shower to rinse off the shampoo from my skin.

Two sad announcements at support group last night. A woman I've never met died from scleroderma over the summer. The accidental death of a young woman's husband was more sobering; he was with her at our June meeting. We were sad for her grief and the grief of their families. Maybe this reminder of life's unpredictability encouraged our opening up about our own lives. Our director, who keeps the conversation flowing, has a way of sharing her story that encourages others to speak. Although the stated theme was nutrition, she let the more pressing emotional issues rule the day.

Thursday, August 14, 2008

Every August, the paternal Italian side of my family has a reunion dinner at the Jersey shore. We toasted my aunt and uncle who could not be there. Uncle could have made the festivities, but Aunt Betty's still sick. A fantastic thunderstorm formed both visual backdrop and soundtrack. Looking out the dining room's windows, I could see the expanse of ocean illuminated intermittently by walls of lightening. My cousin's boys, twelve and eighteen, have grown up kind and charming. The younger held my gift poem close to his face for a long time. In saying goodnight, the boys, young men really, brown from summer with eyes as blue as mine, went around the table giving hugs to each of us. As the wine did its work, the levity increased. At this oceanfront resort and restaurant that caters to Northern Italian-American families, we were the loudest laughing table.

Sunday, September 28, 2008

Today, in the sanctuary of my church home, I was touched by the beauty of the people, seeing them not as a formal congregation sitting in pews, but as a community various in ethnicity, economics, education, age, and lifestyles. Led by a pastor who is self-effacing, with mostly appealing imperfections and a great sense of humor.

Thursday, October 2, 2008

The support group distracted me from the week's worries. There was the initial go-around and socializing. Ways to control Raynaud's. All agree, the change from summer to fall/winter, and from winter/spring to summer is difficult.

There's a medication for Raynaud's out, a hand gel containing nitroglycerin.

Such respect and care these people have for one another. Although we're a group including strangers, I believe we're becoming part of each other's healing networks.

Thursday, November 26, 2008

For fifteen Thanksgivings, I've remained an accepted member of Bob's extended family. We get together almost every month. Any statesman's or family member's birthday is sufficient excuse to gather. Usually I contribute salad, string beans with sliced almonds, or guacamole (made from scratch, of course). One of the grandchildren might read a printout of a humorous tale from the Internet. Bob's first wife's yeoman service as the main cook is central. Table talk's relaxed and covers the gamut from work and health concerns to the food on our plates. Even politics is a fair subject for a group with mainly harmonious views.

Thursday, December 4 2008

I'd arranged for our scleroderma support group to hold the holiday dinner in my building because the hospital where we usually meet had no available space. Telephone began ringing before midafternoon, the co-op's manager telling me that the decorators and caterers are supposed to use the back entrances. They'd already entered from the front.

Our director, who's been dealing with a family emergency this week, stayed for the entire evening, greeting and caring for each guest, true in her commitment to the Foundation and to us. The tables were decorated with small gifts for each guest and a separate table was piled high with presents given away as "prizes." I'm continually impressed with the work of the volunteers. The food, some catered and some prepared by the group, was delicious. A handful of children, two years old and older, came with their parents to honor family members living with scleroderma, or those who have passed on.

A singing group from the university provided lively entertainment. Their willingness both to engage us and to tell about themselves brought genuine cheer.

Saturday, January 24, 2009

For Bob, his knighting service was a complete surprise. For the guests, about twenty of us, it was a game we agreed to play together in celebration of his landmark birthday. The late-afternoon sun shone through the windows of the blue-and-white chapel interior. Nathalie and I had hung a British flag high in the chancel. We had placed, front and center, an antique sword on a low table with a pillow for Bob to kneel on. Thank God, when the moment came, he was able to kneel.

Ten minutes before the ceremony, two friends played baroque tunes on their recorders. At three o'clock, a member of The Madrigal Choir rang a brass bell three times. That was the cue for the "Herald" at the back of the chapel to call everyone to rise for the entrance of the "Queen." The new pastor of the church processed, following the tall stout bagpiper all rigged out for the occasion. Next, the "Herald" entered in his Cambridge doctoral robes. At last, the "Queen" walked slowly down the aisle, wearing a pale-green suit and a rather large black hat. She waved her little wave and smiled that little smile in perfect imitation of England's queen.

Thursday, February 5, 2009

Exercised and napped so I could be alert at our support group meeting. Attendance was larger than usual. The executive director of our region announced her upcoming retirement, promising to attend meetings and stay connected.

Tonight's theme: the psychological impact of scleroderma. We watched an eight-minute film in which Dr. Lee S. Shapiro conducted patient interviews. He and the interviewees spoke about what had been most helpful in managing physical symptoms as well as promoting a sense of general well being. During the subsequent discussion, we made a list what contributes to our psychological balance. Support from our physicians and families, our religious communities, and journaling received the highest votes.

Friday, February 27, 2009

The counseling ministry's clinical director called this morning in response to my letter considering a six months' notice of retirement. He asked me to think about staying on with a loosening of my contract, which includes fewer hours, a pay adjustment, and time off in winter. By staying, I could be at home in the mornings and see clients a couple of afternoons a week. By leaving, I would lose my close relationship with staff, and my long-term spiritual direction clients who, after four or five years, contribute as much to my spiritual walk, perhaps, as I to theirs.

Wednesday, March 18, 2009

Got up early to drive to the little Lutheran church where, for almost eighteen years, I've served intermittently as celebrant and co-celebrant for the early weekday service. Just a few more than a handful present. The liturgy's by heart, no paper or books to hold. We read a Psalm; we hug one another during the passing of the peace. If one sits in the chair to ask for healing for oneself or someone else, the others put a hand on the person's head or back. At the end, the sign of the cross is drawn with oil on each forehead.

Thursday, April 2, 2009

A rheumatologist I've never met was guest speaker tonight at the support group meeting. Arriving late, I grabbed a bottle of water and sat up close to the projection screen. I could see participants having a hard time with the avalanche of medical terms. I was trying to write everything down before the next "power point." Wish presenters would begin by offering a glossary of the less familiar terms they'll be using. Later, a dental hygienist in our group confessed to me how confused she was by the speed and complexity of the presentation.

Felt emotionally cut off tonight for the first time. At my late arrival, there was no operating leader. Pizza, cookies, and water had been placed on the darker side of the room. We were sitting too far apart. The immense conference tables separated us from one another like islands.

Sunday, April 5, 2009

Although still weak from my procedure a few days ago, felt compelled to attend the inter-religious service. This evening's gathering was intended to begin the community's healing from the tragic loss of lives from Friday's shootings in our city. Over a thousand people crowded the school auditorium. Comfort was offered in the prayers of priests, rabbis, and imams. Two boys from a mosque sang hauntingly beautiful chants.

After an hour, the air in the auditorium was hot and stale. Relief came by way of young Muslim women wearing full-length dresses and head coverings. The one who served our section was dressed all in white. In Islam, is white clothing a symbol of mourning? The women went around the auditorium from to row to row, offering bottles of spring water and tissues. In this miniature world of Christians, Jews, Muslims, and unidentified others, at a time when our community was hurting and bereft, their gesture seemed an example of Divine Love.

Chapter 8
FRIENDS, NEIGHBORS, PETS

"Friendship is a sheltering tree."

~Samuel Taylor Coleridge

Many young people move away from their hometowns. Sometimes we may wonder about our old friends from childhood, the people we grew up with. I have stayed in close touch with one friend, Nathalie. We have attended most of our high school reunions and noticed, as the years went by, a softening of personalities and hearts. In our class of less than one hundred students, a few died young; a number were touched by tragedy. We can recall details, like a star of our school's football team who developed heart trouble and went back to college to become a teacher, and the girl we voted "most beautiful" who was absent from every reunion we can remember. At the last two events, everyone wore nametags so we could recognize each other. Yet, even now with our inevitable physical changes, there is a way in which we are still the neat kids we used to be.

To make new friends when age or sickness intervenes is not easy; however, as long as one can get out the door to see a few of the same folks a couple of times a week, a person is almost destined to form new friendships. The most vital groups seem to be those involved in helping others, or those where a new discipline or skill is learned and/or practiced together.

For people with SSc cold weather may be the biggest deterrent to visiting, volunteering, or working outside the home. Living with others in a community setting has the potential for in-house relationships. I live in a cooperatively owned building. Even on days that are beastly cold, when no one ought to venture outside—at least no one with Raynaud's, sensitive lungs, or some form of arthritis—there are many neighbors content to stay at home. Every shared space is a potential meeting place: the pool, the exercise room, the mail room, the laundry room, even the elevator during certain hours of the day. Nearly everyone greets everyone else. Neighbors become acquaintances. Acquaintances become friends as we begin to grow in concern for one another.

One day, having just returned from vacation, I was surprised by a hug in the elevator. The next morning another neighbor hugged and kissed me, in the pool! As a recovering introvert, I must confess I've begun to enjoy, participate, and look forward to these unexpected gestures of affection.

Cultivating close friendships may be a higher priority for single persons than for those living with a spouse, partner, or family members. Even though intimates may provide a social comfort zone, friends of all ages and backgrounds can enliven our days. Acquaintances and co-workers can offer new perspectives, sometimes propping up our dreams better than those who know us best. Slowly or quickly, over years or days, someone we work with, or swim with, or walk with, or sit next to on the patio, may become a meaningful part of our lives.

Pets can become trusted friends and companions. Whether or not you have difficult health issues, a dog or cat, bird, or other creature can offer the reassuring presence of a living, breathing being.

Friday, May 9, 2008

What a great reunion! Nathalie arrived with arms full of lilacs. I set a beautiful table with china and crystal. We talked continually even while we ate, the way we always do when we first get together. After a couple of hours, we calm down and hang out. We had pasta for "dessert" with oil and garlic, highlighting her gift of exquisite parmesan we grated at the table. Garlic's a heavy-duty spice, but I have excuses for celebrations.

Saturday, May 10, 2008

Stirrings in the kitchen around 8:30 a.m.; Nathalie already drinking her coffee. Her suitcase contains not merely clothing and other essentials, but organic coffee beans and a hand grinder and, this time, a pile of her old piano pieces, scores she had not touched since she was a music student forty years ago.

Her hours of playing this morning were a delight to hear, providing background for my work at the computer in the next room. At noon we went out to meet Bob for lunch, then came back to rest and prepare to attend an art show.

Tuesday, June 10, 2008

Some dreams fall into the category of unconscious gold. Last night's was one of them.

I was sitting next to the man who's been my counseling supervisor for five years. In the fifteen years before, he was first, my teacher, then, my spiritual director. We've always kept within the boundaries of our professional roles, yet I've always thought of him as a friend. He is the sort of human being who retains the essence of "friend" in every role.

The dream: We were sitting side by side, holding hands tightly while watching people file by, strangely varied people. Each person paused, looking first into his eyes, then into mine, and afterwards, disappeared into the distance. Some in the procession had a glow about them, as if infused by light. One man's veins were illuminated from beneath his skin in red and blue, the way the body's circulatory system appears on medical wall charts. Many had expressions of hurt in their eyes. They engaged each of us silently, as though attempting to communicate, and moved on.

Waking, I felt deep comfort. My friend and I had been able to support one another during a visit to an unknown realm. We had conferred with extraordinary beings, wordlessly. After falling asleep again, I entered the same dream a second time, with the same characters, the same amazement on waking, and the same deep comfort.

Most dreams are like the first draft of a writing assignment. My impulse, usually a good one, is to throw the thing into the trash. This one's for keeping. Occasionally, in the fabric of a dream, I discover the key to something hidden. I'm asking now: "What door does this dream open?"

Confronting an extraordinary situation with my teacher/supervisor and, by extension, my "better self" suggests I'll always have a trusted confidant: a person, a self, with whom it is safe to confront disturbing mysteries. What is the best a teacher, a spiritual director, or a supervisor, can give? Safe support, quiet wisdom, clear direction, an example of steadiness when life gets shaky.

Not only in the world of dreams but in our everyday lives, disturbing mysteries appear. Autoimmune diseases, including scleroderma, can change the way we see ourselves and others. Sometimes they even can change the way we look. For such a journey, we need a trusted guide.

Thursday, July 31, 2008

Friends I haven't seen in years, Ray and Retta, arrived this morning. We cheerfully spent an entire day together. We ate. We laughed. We reviewed our recent health histories. A spectacular keyboard musician, Retta used to play the organ in a church I served. We looked at photographs, and took some. We talked politics. We caught up on our life and work interests. Recently, Ray received recognition for his continuing ministry of support and assistance to persons with HIV and Aids, a ministry he credits me with inspiring while I was his pastor.

Some sweet moments when we took a break after lunch. Roy dozed on the living room couch while Retta played the piano, the notes flowing from memory. Giving in to my predictable fatigue, I lay down on my bed in the adjoining room and let the sounds wash over me. Music, like friendship, is a healing thing.

Friday, August 1, 2008

Barbara showed up for breakfast before eight. She emits pure energy like a child who never stops moving from place to place. She was the dazzle to my morning reticence—her shirt and jacket, electric blue. I, in my dark stripes, was a little slow in finding the jar of milk, the right knife to cut the apples. Maybe this is the best way for us to visit: talk, laugh, eat, and hug goodbye.

Reviving my youthful shyness about stimulating people and events, I no longer have to dazzle; too much dazzling, from either side, may be injurious to my health.

Sunday, September 1, 2008

Relaxing evening. Bob's great-grandchildren jumping around, and his grandsons, gently awkward in their newly adult bodies provided recreation for the day. After dinner, we played Trivial Pursuit. This game we play at every family gathering offers a backdrop, a kind of ritual structure, for us to enjoy one another, to share our lives. At center stage, a charming four-year-old, Bob's great-granddaughter, has just learned to throw the dice. These people are my cherished crossover of family to friends, friends to family.

Wednesday, October 9, 2008

Sang with an ensemble from The Madrigal Choir at Temple, and followed along in the prayer book with the congregation for several hours without a break. Yom Kippur is the time Jews are encouraged to ponder the theme of confession and forgiveness. There's healing in forgiveness. Rabbi Jesus taught the same truth. Today's rabbi suggested we think of people in our lives with whom we need to reconcile.

In my twenties, anxious and immature, I ended my marriage when our son was small. This morning, during the service, I made an inward vow to apologize to my son's father in person when we meet next week in California. The broken relationship with my sister I've tried, and failed, to restore. During this long day of singing and contemplation, I vowed inwardly to write or call, to try again.

Monday, November 17, 2008
    I'm worried about Bob. His respiratory illness is lasting too long.

Having close friends for the journey sometimes requires letting them be. Dehydration may be part of his problem; he hates drinking water. Type-2 diabetes and one kidney have not slowed his regular indulgence in chocolate, coffee, and a weekly platter of I what I call "manufactured fried clams," clam strips that appear to have been spit out of a plastic manufacturing machine directly into a batter for frying.

My concern for him has altered Bob's lifestyle choices only slightly. He's either lucky or surrounded by a band of guardian angels. Hope his luck holds out and the angels stay.

Sunday, December 14, 2008
    Went to the church where I last served, to see the Christmas pageant. Cranky from the winter cold, I was impatient with the adolescent shepherds; then, with the angels who, having fulfilled their roles seemed to hang around overlong at the manger. I identified with the shy, soft spoken Black Virgin Mother. Cheer came by way of the littlest children-- all lambs, crouched, silent, in a row along the edge of the scene, holding hand-crafted sheep masks up to their faces. Afterwards, parishioners whom I hadn't seen for a long time hugged me. One gave me a bouquet made from altar flowers. All in all, despite the early chill, this turned out to be an unexpectedly good Advent morning.

Thursday, January 22, 2009

I'm excited. My two closest friends' birthdays are today, different years. Fresh red carnations and little UK flags for Bob's upcoming knighting party are already in vases in my office, ready for Saturday's service in the chapel. Nathalie's arriving this afternoon to help. Washed her bedding including a quilt to put over one of my mother's old crocheted afghans so she'll stay warm in the night.

Saturday, February 21, 2009

Marianne rang the doorbell this morning just as I was hanging up from talking with my son.

I met Marianne at a church picnic last summer; she has lupus, lupus erythematosus. Since she is an RN, I expected her understanding of autoimmune diseases to be more complete than mine. Lupus is a close relative of scleroderma, and falls under the specialty of neurology. She warned me that she's an introvert and may not be as forthcoming with information as another person for these conversations. I understand introversion very well.

Immediately on her arrival, I witnessed Marianne's extreme sensitivity to harsh fabrics. She looked carefully around my living room before choosing to sit on the smooth leather couch. When she spoke about her skin sensitivity, I moved decorative textured pillows from the corners of the area near where she sat.

"I think it's neurological," she said, referring to her skin sensitivity.

In short order, I realized how foolish it would be to make generalizations about diseases in the autoimmune family. Marianne has had no upper digestive problems. She described her salad lunches filled with raw vegetables; she does not take vitamins or supplements.

She expressed anger toward some of her physicians who have disbelieved the reality of her pain and other symptoms. Fatigue is a big issue for her. At present, we have in common easily depleted energy banks, and most of our time together we compared notes on overdoing and pacing.

Tuesday, March 24, 2008

I've been putting off being with my closest friends. Most of the last two months consumed with health concerns. This morning, though weak and having to brave the sub-zero temperature, I pushed myself to have breakfast with Lynn. The place was busy, loud, not conducive to conversation. We ate our eggs and pancakes and postponed to a later, warmer time.

At a defensive driving class last winter, Lynn recognized me before I recognized her. She used to refer clients to me at my former counseling agency and we hadn't met or talked for more than a decade. She told me she has multiple sclerosis; I told her I have scleroderma. She agreed to meet to discuss self-care issues.

Wednesday, April 15, 2009

Barbara was respectful of my weakness and fatigue; she didn't seem to notice my dozing off while we poured over a manuscript in her sunny living room.

When Barbara went to the kitchen to make tea, Trouble, the family dog, came up to lick my cheek, pawing me softly. Her sloppy affection roused me, got me to thinking how pets can be contributors to our health. I remember Shep, a collie shepherd mix whose lifeline connected my childhood to my adulthood. After her death, I adopted cats I tried to train as dogs.

Rusty, the smartest of my series of several cats, learned to come indoors when I clapped my hands, but wouldn't roll over even for a piece of raw chicken. After I fully accepted Rusty's feline identity, she became more affectionate, would jump up onto the back of a sofa or chair if I was sad. If I cried, she'd rub her furry back against my face, wiping my tears. Good pets, like good friends, are able to show profound sensitivity.

Unfortunately, the co-op where I live currently excludes all pets but fish, and those uninvited tiny ants that arrive from the patio on my shoes. Each spring, guiltily rethinking Hindu compassion, I buy little round tins of poison to put in the corners of my kitchen floor.

I've considered buying two brightly colored fish, yellow and green; but I don't like the idea of their being locked up in a tank, considering what could go wrong in that environment. I've just about given up my fantasy about getting a green or blue parakeet. My maternal aunt always had a parakeet or two. My grandmother, who kept live parrots, also had a parrot of paper maché after which she named her book of poems.

I have a bird clock. Its electronic chirps and calls make me smile. The realistic cooing of the mourning dove reminds me of childhood summers at my grandparents' shore bungalow.

My bird clock friends run on AA batteries and produce no seed shells, poop, or dropped feathers to clean up. Someday I'm going to write a madrigal about how I love my bird clock. All that ticking and intermittent cooing would make nice cacophony in four-to-six-part harmony.

On the subject of friends, for most of my life, I have paid little attention to their warnings. Colleagues in parish and counseling settings would remark on my symptoms: intermittent sudden significant weight loss, severe muscle and back pain, digestive ills so bad that once I was out of work for a week, scarcely able to swallow water. My former internist kept diagnosing flu; and to be fair, I never mentioned my joint and back pains to him. I took those only to my chiropractor.

A few friends actually suggested I might have a hard-to-diagnose disease. For me, the Raynaud's attacks, frequent coughing and bronchitis, the weak spells, and fatigue were an accepted part of my daily life for as long as I can remember. I had my own diagnostic theories, which included "frostbite" for the red, white, and blue fingers and "reactive depression" for the fatigue. For the "low blood- sugar" weak spells, I stored cheese and yogurt in the staff refrigerator to snack on every couple of hours.

Now and then my family asked how I was doing. But they continued to think what they have always thought, that I am a sensitive plant not particularly adaptable to living in the world. The repetition of symptoms drew a repetition of responses.

"You're too thin," my mother would say, "and you do too much." And she was right.

Self-diagnosis can be a dangerous game. Perhaps I ought to have acted on the suggestions of colleagues and my friends to try to get to the bottom of my long-term medical issues. Would I have been diagnosed earlier? My primary physicians had no clue; I was relatively healthy, still am. My yearly blood work results were in the normal range. Still are.

A man in our support group was almost forced to diagnose himself. After having suffered more than a year of debilitating pain, swelling, and stiffness in his hands and, having consulted with several specialists referred by his primary, he searched the Internet, correctly identifying his condition as the diffuse form of scleroderma. Those specialists to whom he had been referred did not include a rheumatologist; all were unfamiliar with SSc. This is a sad commentary on the lack of awareness about systemic scleroderma in both general and specialized medicine.

Chapter 9
READING, WRITING, AND THINKING

"Whenever you are fed up with life, start writing: ink is the great cure for all human ills, as I have found out long ago."

~C.S. Lewis, from The Letters of C.S. Lewis to Arthur Greeves

Journaling has been the most valuable tool for evaluating where I stand in relation to my illness, as well for dealing with the fallout from various setbacks. Julia Cameron's *The Artist's Way* (Tarcher, 1990) motivated me to commit to this discipline. Cameron incorporates the importance of self-care in developing creative gifts, and recognizes the role our unconscious life plays in the process of learning to reach beyond our perceived limitations.

Monday, June 9, 2008

Spent time this afternoon reading *Breakthroughs in Arthritis* by Thomas MacPhearson Brown, M.D (M. Evans and Company, 1993). The book promotes the theory that SSc is a treatable infection, as are certain forms of arthritis. His success with long-term antibiotic therapy has resulted in apparent cure, or extended remission, for a significant percentage of people diagnosed with SSc.

The first question I have is about the antibiotic. How would taking a drug such as Tetracycline, even a low dosage, for up to a period of two years affect intestinal flora? The FDA and the NIM have not approved this treatment for arthritis-related diseases, which may be the reason rheumatologists won't touch it with a ten-foot pole. An acquaintance reported she and her friend traveled to a Boston physician who continues to practice Brown's therapy. She claims both were cured of their scleroderma as proven by follow-up negative ANA tests. At this news, her rheumatologist told her she probably did not have scleroderma in the first place.

Friday, June 13, 2008

Been thinking about my message for Sunday: "Healed and Healer." Here's a truth no one can fathom: How do the physician, the sick person, and the Source of all Good, by which I mean God, meet in the exchange we call the healing event?

Scleroderma is not the only disease where process and progress are greatly individualized; every disease develops uniquely in every patient. I hope by knowing my own body, its weaknesses and changing needs, I might be better equipped to select or reject recommended treatments from the fields of both traditional and alternative medicine.

Wednesday, June 18, 2008

Told my internist about the woman who tested positive for scleroderma in one of our local laboratories, and again in Boston before beginning treatment with doctors practicing Brown's "breakthrough" in arthritis treatment.

After undergoing treatment, this woman claimed she tested negative for scleroderma on the ANA test, and reported a similar outcome for her friend, a younger woman, who had had a more advanced case, including ulcerated fingertips. After long-term treatment with a form of Tetracycline, the woman I know reported no further joint pain. She said her friend had no further disabling Raynaud's attacks, therefore, no finger ulcers. I don't know what to make of this testimony, or of her rheumatologist's response in which, allegedly, he reversed his initial diagnostic assessment.

My open-minded internist told me that most people have little or no reactivity toward the drug. I guess he was telling me: in diseases where is no conclusive medical solution, one can choose to experiment with alleged cures.

Cures heard and read about, especially those that have not reached mainstream medicine, demonstrate how differently individuals deal with the issue of incurable illness. *Lorenzo's Oil* is a film dramatization of an Italian couple whose young son was diagnosed with ALD, a rare incurable disease. Doctors predicted that he would die before reaching puberty. Neither the child's mother nor his father had advanced education, yet they researched and experimented tirelessly until they were able to create a remedy in a base of olive oil. There was no interference by corporate interests, no medical politics. The parents' passion to preserve their son's life was their sole motivation. The child Lorenzo grew to be a man; he died at age thirty, his mother having pre-deceased him.

Tuesday, July 1, 2008

Stopped by the Scleroderma Foundation office. Picked up a book recommended by my Albany specialist: *Perspectives, Living with Scleroderma* (The Scleroderma Foundation, Inc. Peabody, Mass., 1997) by Mark Flapan. The author, a psychologist, died before he could personally edit his writings for the book. Dr. Flapan was central to the formation of the Scleroderma Foundation and used his considerable skills to help people suffering from this disease.

Also, borrowed the second edition of *The Scleroderma Book, A Guide for Patients and Families,* by Maureen D. Mayes, M.D. (Oxford University Press, 2005). I've had the first edition from the year of my diagnosis. Mayes' provides clear descriptions of the range of symptoms and treatments for the various forms of scleroderma. Her chapter on the relationship of doctor and patient notes the importance of diagnostic testing and personal medical information keeping. She wisely presents some of the mildest as well as some of the most serious case examples of patients with scleroderma.

Wednesday, July 23, 2008

This week's chaplains' retreat lectures disappointing because the presenter hardly touched on subjects of stress and disease. The content was doggedly reminiscent of my psychology courses. The most engaging variation on the Body and Soul theme was today's exercise in which each of us wrote a letter to our body. After surviving the silliness of the idea, I thought a long time and wrote many drafts, trying to answer these questions: How do I speak to my physical self: in what tone, to what purpose, with how much awareness? Is there tenderness in my voice? Is there accusation? Is there humor?

Tonight's session involved participant's statements around the theme: "Why is it so hard to take care of myself?" A woman, serving as chaplain in a mental health setting revealed she has multiple sclerosis and told how, at the onset of the disease thirty years ago, she lost her vision. She believes negative stress in her personal life may have contributed to bringing on her illness. As she became more intentional about self-care, especially by removing herself from toxic relationships, her health returned. Although the changes she made are not easily quantifiable, and she still has "the disease," she walks without a cane and has fully regained her sight.

Friday, August 29, 2008

Tonight I read to the halfway point in the 2005 edition of Mayes' *The Scleroderma Book.* I'm not surprised that predisposing genes as well as environmental factors may contribute to the development of SSc. Environmental factors include chemicals, food and drink, air pollutants, among others. I see on the scleroderma website Dr. Mayes is heading up a research project on the study of genetics in scleroderma. Except for a second cousin on my father's side diagnosed with Epstein Barr, there is no known history of autoimmunity in my family.

To fully participate in the process of our own healing, we may need to sharpen our awareness of reactivity to certain foods, medications, and chemicals. Important, too, may be our reactions to people or events that disturb our psychological and spiritual balance. A heightened consciousness may lead us to make adjustments in our self-care no doctor may think to recommend.

While we may gain insight about how to encourage the healing process in ourselves or in others, we cannot control this process. Nor can doctor, shaman, or priest. The healing agent may speak the word of life, provide the healing ointment, soothe the pain. He or she may cut away diseased tissue and prescribe medication or treatments to assist in the body's restoration. As for the power that knits the wound together, I must confess the God answer.

Tuesday, September 23, 2008

An article in the local paper today cites "resetting the immune system" or stem cell surgery for people with scleroderma. Years may go by before such a procedure is widely available. Stem cell research, which is the basis of many hoped-for cures, is easier to defend politically in patients with SSc because cells are taken from the patient's own body.

Friday, November 7, 2008

Here at the American Association of Pastoral Counselors regional conference, I've been tuning into the lectures by Pamela Cooper-White, PhD, author of *Shared Wisdom: Use of the Self in Pastoral Care and Counseling* (Fortress Press, Minneapolis, MN, 2004) and *Many Voices: Pastoral Psychotherapy in relational and theological perspective* (2007). Paring my notes way down, I'm left with this distillation:

A practitioner who views himself or herself as the sole agent of healing may not be able to be with the patient in a way that frees the patient to believe in the multiplicity of healing possibilities, or to choose from them wisely. Likewise, the patient who sees the practitioner as the sole agent of healing may be held back from initiating self-care practices, or believing what she or he does or does not do might make a difference in her/his health or longevity. Inviting God into the dyad of physician and patient implies there is a shared Power coming from a different Being, a different Place. The thinking of Jewish theologian Martin Buber supports this.

>Thursday, February 12, 2009
>Some days I've a sense the world's becoming a sorrier place. The rich feel threatened by new administration's vow to try to promote fairer distribution of money and opportunity. From a global perspective, I guess I'm rich, since I manage about as well as I did before the financial downturn; but I don't think of change as a threat. For things to get better, everyone must make intentional changes if our planet is to survive.

>Monday, March 2, 2009
>This morning I was wondering about the stories of Jesus' healings. They are remarkable partly for the apparent speed with which the Nazarene worked.

I'm thinking more now about the speed with which we attempt to understand Jesus', or any other healer's interventions. Slowing down brings new clarity to my perceptions; and my experience of healing, in myself and in folks I know, has usually taken time. The word of healing is swift; the process that follows requires persistence and a fresh awareness within the recipient, which can come at a high cost.

As a young woman I read descriptions of Edgar Cayce's recommendations for applications involving of castor oil. Castor oil has proven to restore not only badly damaged skin cells, but diseased cells underneath the skin. In my thirties, I began to apply castor oil regularly, meditatively, to the skin of my entire body. I had suspicion of a malady which, I am certain, involved intuition about my both psychological and physical vulnerabilities.

In Cayce's *Circulating Files on Scleroderma*, there are detailed records of two women he treated over a period of years. Each appeared to be suffering from acute onset of the diffuse type of the disease. After years of work with Cayce, each enjoyed a remarkable recovery. His methods are still being used by individuals; and books and articles documenting results of his treatments and thinking are still being printed and catalogued by the Association of Enlightenment and Research in Virginal Beach.

A personal note: After my mother was diagnosed with diabetes-related kidney failure, her doctor prescribed dialysis. She requested time to consider. For a week she stayed at my parsonage while I administered castor oil packs daily to her kidney area. She never followed up on the doctor's order for dialysis. My mother lived the next seven years, after the onset of her blindness, in a residential nursing home where castor oil was applied to her kidney area after her baths. While her attendants did not apply the packs strictly according to Edgar Cayce's guidelines, and may not have been aware of the importance of this treatment, I have always believed continuation of the oil rubs prolonged my mother's life. The next time she refused dialysis, she was ready to die.

I am not recommending that any person with kidney failure refuse dialysis in favor any experimental alternative treatment. I do realize there may have been a mistake in the evaluation of the seriousness of my mother's condition, or even a monumental placebo effect with regard to the applications. However, I do wonder if a person with some fear, or prediction, of compromised kidney function may not benefit from the application of castor oil packs as preventive therapy.

Wednesday, April 15, 2009

With every massage, my therapist teaches me a new phrase referring to an anatomical site. The area around the scapula is called "pillars of hope." These non-medical terms she learned during her training at The Finger Lakes School of Therapeutic Massage. It's a fine day when the medical and poetic can exist side by side for the good of the whole organism, like the two sides of a well-functioning brain. The "pillars of hope" location is where we place our hand when giving sigh of relief, or grief; the place we touch when we say: "God willing!"

Chapter 10
THE BASICS

Food/Exercise/Sleep

"Think in the morning, act in the noon, sleep at night."

~William Blake

We have freedom to make individual choices about what we eat, how we move, and the amount, and sometimes the quality, of sleep we get. We also are free to follow our physicians' recommendations and take our prescribed medications, or not. The amount and quality of water we drink may contribute to our healing. In most parts of the world, pure water is not free; however, in the West, most can afford to filter tap water, or purchase spring or purified water in multi-gallon glass containers.

The basics are deceptively simple, yet there can be pitfalls if we rely on them to solve all our health issues. This past year's medical events led to radical changes in my diet. Clearly, I made numerous missteps along the way.

Also, my self-prescribed exercise routine produced no increase in bone density; in fact, my bone density decreased. The pain and weakness in hip and knee, which included mild atrophy, were unresponsive to chiropractic treatments. However, a course of physical therapy prescribed by my local rheumatologist corrected both pain and motility problems, at least temporarily. I exchanged the stationary bike and rowing machines for a twice- a-week weight-bearing class.

Sleep, so necessary to general health and well-being, has been my friend, mostly; although pain from reflux was a serious problem for years. Many things can interfere with a good night's sleep. If sleep apnea is suspected and a sleep test confirms this, a C-PAP device may be prescribed. This is a mask that regulates breathing and should make way for safer, deeper sleep. Some people have a difficult time adjusting to the C-PAP. Fit and sleep position need to be taken into consideration. For those with latex allergies, be aware that there are elastic straps that hold the device in place on the face. These may need to be replaced with a non-latex alternative.

In SSc, as in other systemic diseases, pain and itching are common reasons for wakefulness. So, also, are stress and worry. Consulting with professionals about both the physiological and the psychological reasons for sleeplessness is a good idea. Yet, however carefully one may follow the doctor's recommendations, or disciplined we may be about diet and exercise, trying to control sleep quality is a tricky business. A loved one in the same bed or room, a child or children who may wake in the night, worries and responsibilities we cannot postpone, all insure our sleep will be interrupted from time to time.

Many people take sleep medications nightly. I would try everything else before resorting to pharmaceuticals as a permanent remedy for sleeplessness. Psychological reasons are usually treatable. Counseling may bring to light not only causes of the worry but, as a bonus, may help resolve disturbing personal issues, whether or not they are related to scleroderma. Bodily renewal is the primary objective for getting quality sleep; and dreaming, often underrated, can help promote this goal by expressing submerged feelings.

There is widespread resistance to eating the "right" foods, following a disciplined exercise program, and preserving conditions for a good night's sleep. Why are we so reluctant to make these lifestyle changes? Here are few of the excuses I've used:

"It's too much trouble;" "I haven't got time;" and "What if it doesn't work?"

There is no guarantee by sticking to healthful disciplines that those with SSc will feel better than we do now, even if we were able to follow up on every detail of self-care. However, a strong desire to function normally for as long as possible may motivate us to act more often on our body's behalf. Research in the field of systemic diseases grows daily. New medications and other treatments are continually being tested. There is hope from more than one source. The ways we are able to care for our own bodies may turn out to be as important as the hoped-for cure beyond the horizon.

Most people take for granted their ability to eat, chew, digest, walk, care for home and family, drive, work, stay awake at meetings and family gatherings, and enjoy occasional travel or entertainment away from home. Those who live in the shadow of a systemic disease cannot take anything for granted. The things we would like to do may be endless. The things we are able to do, as time goes on, may become severely limited.

The following journal entries are anecdotal. They provide snapshots of my mistakes as well as what I hope are helpful insights. A self-care plan for every individual needs to be worked out in conversation with trusted medical professionals. This documentation of my process is intended primarily to motivate readers to keep records of their own.

FOOD

Thursday, May 8, 2008

I love breakfast. I'm steeping a cup of green tea. Cream of buckwheat, my favorite cooked cereal with ground flaxseed sprinkled over the top, already in the bowl. Sprouted grain toast with a thick layer of almond butter or goat cheese will be my hit of protein.

I'm hoping the new calcium citrate and vitamin D will make up for what I may be losing from possible blocking of nutrients by my medications. B 12 also has become more difficult for me to absorb. For some people, eating the foods that contain these nutrients is enough to keep up normal blood levels; but regular testing for B 12, calcium and D levels convinced me I require supplementation. My chiropractor's guiding me in my choice of food-based vitamins. We're moving slowly with this so that we can see how I tolerate each substance. In vitamins and supplements, as in drugs, one size does not fit all.

My first real memories of food began at age eight. My stepfather had just married my mother and moved us from our city row home to a one-family house in the fresh country air. Year round we ate vegetables from our backyard garden as they ripened, and all through the winter as the product of my mother's home canning. Whole milk and cream were delivered from the dairy to our doorstep. A flock of Rhode Island Reds inhabited a large fenced yard and were cooped at night in our second garage, providing eggs and poultry for our table year round.

After my stepdad retired, we went for whole summers to Sebago Lake, Maine, where we ate lobsters and clams steamed over a driftwood fire on the sand. The water from the springs that fed the lake was pure. While out in the little fishing boat, we drank from metal cups dipped straight into the lake. There was a water pipe that extended along the lake floor; a pump in the boathouse sent the water directly up the hill to our faucets. With all this natural living, how did I go wrong?

Friday, May 16, 2008

Woke up this morning with a swollen right eyelid, which years ago I named "sugar eye." When, over a few days, I've eaten more refined sugar than my body can tolerate, a small amount by most standards, swelling forms under my eyelid. Even too much fresh fruit may lead to "sugar eye." Twice in my thirties, a "sugar eye" turned into a crusty cyst under my lid called a chalzion that had to be surgically removed. Eliminating my intake of sweets, soaking my lids under a warm, moist compress, and applying a warm, wet teabag at the first sign of redness has kept me from a recurrence of the chalzion. My former chiropractor thought I might be allergic to sugar. What does this have to do with scleroderma?

Even if peculiar only to me, this eye symptom creates a question about how amounts and types of sugar in the diet might impact persons with SSc and other autoimmune diseases.

Tuesday, May 20, 2008

On this busiest day of the week, I order my regular takeout of tofu, shrimp, and bok choy. No matter how carefully I explain to the English-speaking host, the Chinese cook still makes mistakes in my order. I end up stir-frying the whole thing again at home in sesame oil with a little fresh garlic and ginger. If I stopped taking the PPI, would I have to give up all spices? Ought I to give them up even while taking the PPI? The drug seems not minimize the incidence of reflux at night.

Tuesday, May 27, 2008

Running from work to chores, to supper, didn't get home until 8:00 p.m., with wicked indigestion. Bob and I went to an Italian restaurant. Bad choice. Although I tried to go light on the tomato sauce, I'm in trouble. A sip of Bob's beer was one sip too many. Am paying dearly.

Monday, June 16, 2008

The air is heavy, humid. Interested to see if the new rose hips vitamin C in two doses, at one and 6:00 p.m. will decrease the swelling in my hands, which appears more related to arthritis than sclerodacktyly. The right hand's most painful in the morning when I first get up.

Sunday, August 24, 2008

Today I began a five-small-meal-a-day experiment. After making more than an hour of telephone calls, I made a fourth meal of a blended yogurt and banana drink. At 8:00 p.m., I'm free from all forms of digestive distress. My internist told me to begin tomorrow to resume taking 15 mgs. of the PPI; and gradually add nutritional supplements, such as calcium and a protein powder, since my worst symptoms seem to have disappeared.

Wednesday, September 4, 2008

I may never again eat at our co-op's social events. Last night's Spiedie Fest was a disaster. A "spiedie" is a Southern Tier of New York creation in which lamb, chicken, or pork is marinated in oil, vinegar, and spices, grilled on skewers, and rolled up in a piece of white Italian bread.

Not one item on the long table of highly spiced, oily, fried, and sugar-loaded foods could pass as easily digestible. Even the salad dressing sent out a tantalizing smell of vinegar and garlic. Giving in, I ate a little of everything. Tasted fine; I'm thinking, "maybe it's all in my head, after all." The final suicide attempt was the consumption of an immense chocolate cookie. This act motivated partly by my desire to show my appreciation to the professional baker who is a co-op neighbor and friend, and partly wanting to deny my reactivity to so many common foods.

Hounded by gastric misery, I finally got to sleep after midnight while propped in a sitting position. From now on, I'll bring my own or stay home.

Monday, October 6, 2008

By suppertime, I was so frustrated with attempting to eat conservatively; I considered taking a double dosage of my PPI in the morning and having two slices of pepperoni pizza for lunch.

Friday, November 7, 2008

On our way to the regional convention, my associate turned into a great homemade ice cream place. The creamy vanilla cone impaled with hunks of chocolate, like all sin, was temporarily exhilarating. I kept subsequent misery to myself.

Friday, December 12. 2008

I've begun treating the beginning of a "sugar-eye" inflammation with tea bags and warm compresses. No more cookies.

Friday, January 9, 2009

Multiple small meals leave me feeling hungry. I'm losing weight. Tried adding a low-sugar dessert and small glass of milk in the midafternoon. Noticed loose bowel symptoms a few hours after. Think it's the milk.

Tuesday, February 17, 2009

At lunch, reflux got bad when I tried to take my vitamins and supplements. There's definitely more to swallowing problem than spices and the size of my capsules.

Tuesday, March 18, 2009

Lunch was a mild Italian sausage with fennel, brown rice, and a boiled sweet potato. For supper, a bowl of homemade chicken broth, salad, a slice of bread with goat cheese, and some honeydew melon. An embarrassment of riches in the middle of Lent. All this effort toward healing my esophagus and the restoration of lost fat and muscle, but will it work?

Friday, March 20, 2009

As sick of fish, broiled and sautéed, as one can get.

Wednesday, March 28, 2009

Felt weak when I came up from swimming, even after a second breakfast. Bob's been taking me to lunch to relieve me of the burden of cooking. He loves to eat out. We enjoy each other's company, but a problem trying to find wholesome foods. Ordered calf's liver and mashed potatoes today, which I gobbled up like a starving person.

The industrial strength PPI that the doctor says is essential for healing my ulcer doesn't agree with me. My stools are so pale; they look like stools a day or two after swallowing barium. Am I not digesting my food? Could this be why I'm so hungry and staying so thin, while eating so much?

Wednesday, April 1, 2009

Think I got away with having a slice of tomato and some fresh green pepper on my sandwich. Half a chocolate chip cookie, however, created quite a ruckus. A cup of green tea is not as soothing to the gut as chamomile.

Tuesday, April 7, 2009

Body rebelling against the whey and yogurt drink I've been swilling to boost my energy. Whey's a cow milk product. I need to find a substitute.

Sunday, May 2, 2009

Shopped for some alarmingly expensive gluten-free foods in the health food store. Dreaded the search for supper. Gave Bob several portions of chicken and lamb stew I cooked and froze a week ago, before I was warned about glutinous grains. Ended up with sardines on a piece of Millet Flax bread, a side of brown rice with *usabi* plum paste, wickedly bitter stuff.

I'm feeling no triumph in being less fatigued after eliminating gluten and dairy products. This experiment interferes not only with my enjoyment of food at home, but is a huge impediment to restaurant dining. Before gluten-free, I could bring my tiny container of real maple syrup, and put it on the table at the breakfast place. Now I can't eat any pancakes made with wheat flour. Wherever we go, I must draw on my talent for acting and deception. Dinner at a restaurant means packing numerous items, including wheat-free soy sauce, olive oil, and goat feta for the salad; a little container of black olives I've chopped up to add to the broiled fish which will arrive predictably pale and flavorless. Discovering restaurants with special items or menus to accommodate my guidelines is harder than adjusting to the new food plan.

EXERCISE

Thursday, May 8, 2008

Around 6:00 a.m. did my stretching exercises on the living-room floor. A few yoga poses for flexibility. Leg lifts to strengthen my abdomen. This takes about fifteen minutes and relieves stiffness left over from the night.

Saturday, June 14, 2008

Flag Day. Had to rush tidying up because Barbara, my high-energy friend, was scheduled to come by to instruct me in weight-lifting. She telephoned at the last minute, asking to meet at her house instead. After we worked out with the weights, she suggested I consult her personal trainer. Right now, taking on another provider is beyond my imagining. I'll try to be careful, take my time, keep my arms close my body, chin slightly tucked, and use the lighter weights until I'm stronger. Without a friend for company, I fear weight-lifting will be too boring to continue.

Friday, June 20, 2008

A mildly productive day. Went to the pool soon after breakfast; walked around a store for over an hour with less leg pain and fatigue than usual. Muscles are not significantly strengthened from my few weeks of working out. Tonight, rode the stationary bike downstairs, rowed, and then sampled the ski machine, which initially threw me a little off balance.

Tuesday, July 22, 2008

A labyrinth's a circular path designed for meditative walking; this one is made from stones and surrounded on every side by beautiful flowering shrubs. Had to pay attention to follow the intricate bends and turns which take a special kind of balance.

Saturday, September 27, 2008

Last time I danced with abandon was at Bob's college reunion more than ten years ago. Since then, I've been held back physically as well as psychologically. Arthritis, fatigue, muscle weakness, and the fact that I'm no longer as attractive as I used to be, kept me in the chair today at the wedding. I miss dancing. I'd like to be able to dance again.

Wednesday, October 22, 2008

Must have been out of my mind to agree to play touch football with the kids last week. After falling backwards from colliding with a much heavier relation, my shoulder hurts too much to work out. Swimming the backstroke used to be my most comfortable style. Now my neck muscles are too stiff to lift my arms over my head, and there's pain in my left hip when I pull on my compression hose.

Tuesday, November 4, 2008

Leg pain from past few days is gone. Last night worked out after supper. Not sure where to find supervision for my exercises.

Tuesday, February 17, 2009

I've been neglecting exercise because of extreme fatigue and digestive troubles. I miss the stretching, but at a loss about what to do.

Sunday, March 15, 2009

Nearly two weeks since my endoscope procedure; seems, by now, I should be stronger. After three hours of Choir rehearsal, I met my swim buddy. The water felt cooler than usual; the tips of my fingers turned blue which hasn't happened in the pool all winter. The reason may be too little exercise, or maybe weakness from the healing ulcer.

Thursday, April 30, 2009

There's a steep stairway to my bedroom here at the monastery. When I arrived yesterday evening, I leaned heavily on the handrail making several trips to carry up my belongings. Today, going up and down, I'm touching the rail only lightly. All this stair-climbing may be strengthening my hips and legs. I go both ways is at least twelve times a day to go to meals, chapel services, and the bathroom.

Saturday, May 9, 2009

I've been trying to translate my monastery stair-climbing to my co-op where there are two short flights between basement and first floor, as well as back stairways, which are remote from human traffic most of the time. A neighbor's discouraging my backstair-climbing because of the danger of falling on concrete in an isolated area.

SLEEP

Wednesday, May 14, 2008

Woke up this morning feeling tired though I'd had eight hours. Uncharacteristically, sailed off for an extra hour. Nice dreaming about my son when he was seven. We were lying in the sand by the seashore, side by side, his head leaning against my arm. When I woke for the second time, I felt rested, at peace. Sometimes I miss my little boy.

Thursday, June 26, 2008

A rainy day, relief from all the heat. Exercise and lots of sunshine may be improving my sleep.

Thursday, July 17, 2008

Trying to be easier on myself. When I can't keep trucking past 8:00 p.m., I'm learning to sign off without excuses. Early to bed should save an hour in the morning for straightening up the apartment before going out.

Saturday, August 16, 2008

A great sleep in Nathalie's guest room last night with the air conditioning off, just the cool, moist, late-summer air all night long. Waking nice and slowly to the rustle of my long-lost New Jersey oaks. This morning, Nathalie and I agreed we look a decade younger.

Sunday, August 31, 2008

Today began, accidentally, at 4:30 a.m. Completed a list of tasks with such zeal, I had to eat a second breakfast before going to church.

Wednesday, October 8, 2008

Lack of sleep colors everything gray and knocks my whole system out of balance. One of those awful nights that just happens now and then. All I did today was practice the music for Yom Kippur eve. After eating and throwing up lunch, I lay on my bed, calling to cancel each of my afternoon clients. I read *The New Yorker* magazine for a couple of hours and kept down a small soup supper.

About a half hour before when I had to arrive at Temple, I lay down on my bed and fell into a sudden, deep sleep. Thank God, I was already dressed to go: music organized, my coat and gloves folded over a chair in the hall. Woke just in time to make it to the service, totally refreshed. The unexpected nap saved my evening from ruin.

Wednesday, January 7, 2009

Not a snow day, just ice: ice on the roads, ice on the sidewalks, a perfect excuse for canceling our out-of-town staff meeting. Went back to sleep after a night of wakefulness. At 4:00 a.m., took a yellow legal pad to list the things I suspect are keeping me awake. Stretched, prayed, slept, and woke again.

Friday, January 30, 2009

I worked until after 8:00 p.m. last night, with too little winding-down time. All the articles on sleep give advice about quieting the mind before bedtime. At 3:00 a.m., thinking about life, work, the world, mortality in general, and mine in particular just made me wider and wider awake. Even focusing prayerfully on family, friends, the inner light, and even on Jesus himself looking kindly down at me, did not bring me closer to any of them, or succeed in drawing me back into sweet unconsciousness.

Saturday, January 31, 2009

Dreamed last night about my strange soulmate [a man with whom I have a powerful, though platonic, connection] who, by now, has robbed me of years of sleep. Maybe dreams are the best place for us to be. No expectations. No rancor. Reality eluded us from the beginning.

Monday, February 23, 2009

After a great massage, I'm more relaxed than in a long time. Last night's hyper-alertness would be puzzling if I hadn't tried to do so much right before bed. I hate being wide awake when it is time to fold up under the covers.

Saturday, March 14, 2009

The best night I've had in a long time. Even after bathroom breaks and sips of water to soothe my drug-dry mouth and throat, slipped back again and again into peaceful sleep.

Monday, March 23, 2009

A friend and I had planned to swim at 7:00 p.m., rather late for me. Those soft-spoken "angels" that show up now and then with warnings hinted I should skip the pool. They were right. I woke up in the middle of the night, thoughts popping and limbs leaping. Prayed for everyone I could think of. Got up, did some yoga stretches, drank some water, and read the rest of the Gospel of Luke. I had to write down everything on my mind before I could fall asleep again.

Wednesday, March 25, 2009

Woke up at 3:00 a.m., tossed for an hour, suspicious there may be something I'm hiding from myself. Sinking into a meditative state, I began uncomfortably looking at me and my behavior. My self-critique produced the following indictments:

I talk too much; I explain too thoroughly. In my practice, sometimes I work harder than my clients on *their* issues. In social situations, I practically stand on my head to entertain, to make people laugh, to reverse the introversion nobody even knows about. Such efforts waste precious energy.

Wednesday, April 15, 2009

Sleep after a massage is more than sleep.

Tuesday, May 5, 2009

Here I am, near the end of my intentional journaling year, turning in a new direction. I woke rested, still asking questions. I guess there are no answers impervious to change and, as long as I live and breathe, no end to my questions.

Chapter 11
DESPERATION RETREAT

> "Jacob was left alone; and a man wrestled with him until daybreak. When the man saw that he did not prevail against Jacob, he struck him on the hip socket; and Jacob's hip was put out of joint as he wrestled with him. Then he said, 'Let me go, for the day is breaking.' But Jacob said, "I will not let you go, unless you bless me.""
>
> **~Genesis 32: 24-26 (NRSV)**

Jacob would not let go of the man, who is sometimes referred to as an angel, until he blessed him. What about the injury the angel man inflicted on Jacob's hip? I bet Jacob was limping for a while after his night of struggle.

There was pain in my hip and anxiety in my heart even before my contentious angel, Mary, came on the scene. Like Jacob, I knew I needed to go away for a while by myself. This would not be a vacation with family or friends. This would be a bold attempt to invite the Source of being to come a little closer. I needed to find answers to the puzzles of my illness, especially the continuing uproar in my GI tract.

Like Jacob, I was limping in pursuit of my vision. My left hip hurt. I was scared of my medications. I was scared of my food. I had a lump in my left calf and a lump in my throat.

A stranger, an angel, even God in various disguises tends to show up when we are feeling most alone, at the apex of solitary. No assurances as to whether or not the messenger is bringing good or ill, and little opportunity for investigation. It's a now-or-never situation. Calling for immediate rescue, we are virtually drowning. This unknown angel being may be able to help, produce a blessing, at least. In the back of our mind, we can recall the warnings, the logic which might have held us back in the past, when we were surrounded by people ready to protect us:

"Don't' talk to strangers, stupid."

I was desperate. Three weeks after the second endoscope documented the healing of my ulcer, I still couldn't get enough food or rest to overcome my weakness. If the gastroenterologist found no pathology, how come I was still so sick? On the day I was scheduled to leave for the monastery, side effects from the "well-tolerated" medication along with a suspected blood clot in my leg, tempted me to cancel. I persevered.

The women's retreat house turned out to be homey with windows that open out to trees and sky. For the first few days, I was their only guest. The food smelled and tasted great; yet, everything except ripe bananas and herbal tea either provoked my suspicion or challenged my digestion. My emergency store of pomegranate juice and rice protein powder filled me up for about an hour, after which my voracious hunger returned.

To provide a wider context, I will begin before the beginning.

Monday, April 27, 2009

Re: trip to the monastery tomorrow, I'm taking too much stuff. No idea what I'll need. Food, indoor temperature, number of guests—all unknown. I'm still asking myself why I'm going, why I didn't put this off until June. I'm desperate, that's why. Going to the monastery on the mountaintop may be the closest I can get to "Kingdom come."

Tuesday, April 28, 2009

Stopped by my chiropractor's office early this morning to show him the inflamed lump in my calf. He didn't think a blood clot would be so close to the skin, but told me to go see my internist, anyway. An hour later, the lump was given a diagnosis of superficial phlebitis with possible infection in a varicose vein, and I was given a prescription for an antibiotic tablet three-quarters of an inch long.

Drove all the way to the monastery with the car windows open wide for relief from the sweltering spring day. Up the forever-winding hill to the entrance my little car climbed, past grazing sheep among a few shaggy ponies and llamas. Why would they put ponies and llamas together with the lambs? (The larger animals are intended to protect the lambs from being snapped up by coyotes and, as I was informed during my stay, their strategic presence doesn't always work.)

Arriving on time for supper, I was afraid of what supper might be. I was greeted at the kitchen door by the "guest mistress." I could smell fragrant chili she was stirring in a little saucepan. Beef, chili, and cooked tomatoes I've avoided for longer than I can remember. Almond butter and rice cakes along with other items I'd packed in my car were my substitute supper.

The chiropractor called my cell phone around 7:00 p.m. and urged me to stay away from milk products. If I'm having an allergic reaction, my reactivity may be too strong to be to taking the PPI for a while, he said. Neither consulting with my chiropractor nor with my gut has been helpful during the past few weeks. I'm looking for answers from elsewhere.

I love my little room with the "St. Teresa" sign on the door. I remember reading about St. Therese of Lisieux, or Saint of the Little Flowers, as she has been called. Terminally ill in her twenties from tuberculosis, her last prayer was that, after her death, she might send down roses to encourage the downhearted.

The internist prescribed moist heat five times a day. Applied a tiny castor oil pack with heat on my leg lump for half an hour. (My friend Edgar Cayce's idea to include the castor oil.)

Lying on my bed in the dark, listening to the rain, I watched the wind rippling the filigreed spruce trees in continuous prayer.

Wednesday, April 29, 2009

Yesterday's freak warmth has vanished. Today I had to work at staying warm. A full breakfast: bran cereal, banana, tea, and honey from the monastery's bees; two pieces of whole wheat bread with almond butter, raspberry jam; and a Clementine. I was thrilled to see a quart of soy milk on my side of the guest fridge. Gut still unsettled.

My son and I talked on our cell phones as he was driving to work this morning. How he solved a problem with his digestion: stopped drinking quantities of water and other liquids with his meals. I never paid much attention to the teachers of yoga who also recommend abstaining from drink while eating; I guess I choose which behaviors to change based on my relationship to the person who makes the recommendation. I tend to listen to my son.

Took a few sips during dinner to get my enzyme capsule down. Taking calcium citrate powder mixed in applesauce is much easier than swallowing tablets or capsules. After a sensible dinner, I made a big mistake. Went crazy with the desserts laid out on the butcher block in the kitchen—a banana, two homemade cupcakes and a spicy tea.

Leg lump appears less inflamed right after applying the heating pad and oil. Wrapped the leg firmly from ankle to knee with an ACE bandage. The skin over the varicosities appears so fragile; I don't see how I could manage without the heavy compression hose.

People with dry mouth conditions, including *Sjogren's*, must sip water or other liquids with their meals. The choice to eat without drinking is only for those who have enough saliva to chew patiently and well. The complete recommendation includes drinking a glass of water a half hour before eating and/or a half hour afterwards.

Thursday, April 30, 2009

We ate dinner at noon, the guest mistress and me, at the same long table with room for eight or ten guests. We exchanged summaries of our lives and work. On the subject of digestion, she admitted to better results from eating without drinking. We laughed and shared a messy mango. Not much conversation the rest of the day.

My internist left message my blood work was normal. Have to keep cell phones off during the day here to respect the silence. He said as long as there is no breakage in the skin, I can forget about taking the antibiotic prescribed by his colleague for the leg lump. Still applying castor oil and wet heat five times a day for half an hour; the lump looks smaller.

Couldn't get enough to eat tonight, the second day with no poultry or fish except some tiny canned shrimp. The sparse offerings may be part of the contemplative discipline. I'd be happy with black beans and rice. Wish I'd brought tuna or sardines. The salad with vegetable and noodle soup wasn't enough to hold me through the night, and my rice powder is an incomplete protein.

I was sitting alone at the table tonight when Mary arrived. The guest mistress had gone to the store, leaving me in charge of welcoming Mary. Her superior air both fascinated and put me off. She was friendly enough, but there was something elusive in her manner. I watched as she ate the salad and skipped the soup, and I asked if she had already eaten. She said she eats no wheat, dairy, or refined sugars, and has food in her car. There were wheat noodles in the soup. She hinted about having an unspecific autoimmune disease.

I asked which foods Mary was able to eat. She said, quite abruptly, she was too tired from her long drive to talk now;

she needed to rest. Before going upstairs to her room, she suggested I attend the evening service in the chapel.

At little before eight, Mary left for the chapel on foot under threat of a thunderstorm. I offered her a ride in my car, which she refused. The distance to the chapel is less than an eighth of a mile, but my legs hurt too much to walk.

The sanctuary was warm. A monk, who may be the youngest, pulled the rope to ring the bell. The remaining monks, all of them very old, filed in slowly. One inched along with a walker. A few coughed. As they took their places in the round chancel area, the electricity was turned off. The light cast by several tall candles was the only light. Rain started to beat down on the roof.

As the monks began to sing, I began to breathe more easily. These old men since before daybreak had been alternating the tending of sheep with the tending of souls. These old men who had made their entrance coughing and limping, one on a walker, one with a cane, had undergone a transformation within moments of their singing. Through sweet harmony, their age and infirmities disappeared before our eyes. They became young and strong. One played a harp that accompanied their chants. The only spoken words were the Lord's Prayer with the priest's request for protection from evil through the night.

If these crippled, ancient, holy men can be so transformed by merely singing, my idea of finding an answer on this mountaintop may not be so far out.

At the close of evensong, the worshippers, mostly from outside the community followed the monks down a steep stairway to the lower level. We bowed before a colorful life-sized icon of Jesus on a cross between the two thieves. The monks sent up prayers before a white marble statue of Mother Mary holding the baby Jesus in her arms. A pond of memorial candles flickered at her feet.

Mary, my mysterious new acquaintance, was there, too, pale as marble herself. Guests stood as close to the monks as we would ever get. The tallest monk had a sharp nose like my Bob's. A short monk, the one who played the harp, swung a sprinkler of holy water over the whole company with the blessing before we went back to our rooms.

I'm hungry, so hungry. Hope I can fall asleep before ten.

Friday, May 1 2009

Woke up a little after 4:00 a.m. shaky and slightly disoriented. Too early to go down to the kitchen. Trained my thoughts on people in places of famine who feel constant hunger, and prayed myself back to sleep for another hour. Around 5:50 went downstairs and ate fruit and bread and almond butter. Drank my pomegranate juice with the rice protein powder. Went back to sleep at 8:00.

After Mass, feeling as protestant as a sore thumb, I drove to the nearest town, downed an egg, cheese, and bacon sandwich at a fast-food chain. Didn't make me feel better, only fuller. Stopped to buy half a rotisserie chicken, thinking I might slip some meat into last night's leftover noodle soup. Never have experienced such strange, furtive hunger.

Our noon dinner was enhanced by the arrival of the weekend guests, professional women, who come back every year, all of them friendly and quick to laugh. One took me to the birthing area in the barn to see the newborn lambs. Though I know William Blake's poem on the subject by heart, I had never seen a lamb only two days old leap and play so joyfully.

Saturday, May 2, 2009

The sky's finally clearing for my last full day at the monastery. After the first sound sleep of the week, I was especially careful at my solitary breakfast. Slices of gluten-free bread offered from Mary's freezer supply were surprisingly good, toasted. Was sitting in the rocking chair under a window in my little room, working on my computer when she appeared in my doorway. Mysterious Mary, there she was, ready to talk to me, to give the word. My heart skipped a beat.

She arrived at exactly 10:00 a.m., as if we had a real appointment. Glad for a bright day and for feeling rested and tuned in, I invited her to sit in the other chair, turned off my laptop, and opened my notebook. "Gluten-free and dairy-free," she explained, was keeping her alive and well; and may do the same for me. There was, however, a hitch, a warning: I would have to follow a detoxification diet at the start before getting into the rhythm of finding the gluten- and dairy-free foods that agree with me. After the detoxification period I will be free to experiment with other foods, such as sprouted grains, and yogurts. I wrote everything down in my notebook. The items for detox omitted all cow dairy, except probiotic kefir; all hard cheeses including goat cheese; gluten, all forms of corn, oats, barley nuts, soy, eggs, salmon, white potatoes, all flours except buckwheat and rice, all refined sugars, no fruit juices, and few fruits. I asked questions:

"Can I ever have cow-dairy again? Yogurt? Cheese?"

"What's wrong with wild salmon?"

"If I can't eat the white of the white potato, how about the *skin* of the white potato?"

She persevered with polite restraint, while I asked an hour of questions and wrote pages of notes.

After her list of "Thou shalt nots," she began a second, much shorter list, of acceptable vegetables, fruits, fish, meats, oils, and grains. Her recommendations, I realized much later, were not far from Edgar Cayce's teachings with which she seemed well acquainted. He cautions against empty starches for persons with scleroderma, such as white potatoes and white bread, although his work preceded the more specific gluten- and wheat-free solution.

I felt so tired and weak; I feared Mysterious Mary's detoxification diet might do me in.

As if she could read my mind, she began to offer hope. She said I could eat a wider variety of foods after three-to-six months, such as special yogurts, certain gluten-free grains, maybe soy beans, tofu, and organic eggs. The fat in ordinary grocery store eggs, she told me, is different from the fat from properly grain-fed, cage-free chickens. Even with her encouragement, the world seems rife with hidden dangers to my gastrointestinal tract.

Before leaving, she advised me to consult with a naturopathic doctor to work out an individualized plan. As I watched her turn to walk out the door, I had the wild notion to grab her by the foot and say, "I will not let you go unless you bless me!"

I closed the door, put the lists on the dresser and stared out my window onto the green hills. I've loved my St. Teresa's room, conversation with the trees, the monks chanting to heaven. Mysterious Mary's message was already a burden, but a burden to consider. With the bright morning sun shining on my face, I fell asleep on my bed, and woke to the chimes announcing our noon meal.

Still mulling over the issue of trusting the messenger. In the past few days, I've learned Mary is a musician and teacher; she plays the violin, just like my mother. There were times growing up when I didn't trust my mother; although oddly, our relationship seems to have improved since she died. I am put off by Mary's air, her reticence, which conveys a tacit authority. If she is Jacob's angel in female form, or Mother Mary come down to test my spirit, I know I am no match. Either could easily wound me; but unlike Jacob, I could never prevail against such force. I would fail, crumble. I can imagine my mother up there in the company of heaven, setting this all up. My retreat week: Mysterious Mary's arriving while I was alone in the house, this morning's sun breaking through just in time for her visit, and all for the sake of getting me on this tortuous detoxification diet, the purpose being to attain greater health in order, of course, to serve more effectively.

I tried my best to play the game. If Mysterious Mary had somehow been able to assume my mother's nature, I certainly worked hard to gain her approval. At every common meal, I put the same foods on my plate that she put on hers. I kept my distance and did not bother her for information after the first night. When she was ready to teach, I was ready to listen, the perfect student, the perfect child, except for asking too many questions.

After supper I went to the early evening service of chanting with the monks—a little congregation of local people and monastery guests. I was surprised to see the director from the counseling agency where I worked more than ten years ago. I sat next to him to in order to share one of the last available Psalm books. During the years I counseled in his agency, we had many disagreements. Tonight, though, we chanted side by side companionably until I was deeply calmed and at one with my true self.

Back in my room, alone, still caught up in the hypnotic chant Mind, I listen for the cue, so I might follow the next tune of praise or supplication. My initial urge to reject Mysterious Mary's recommendations is softening. Her gluten-free toast did taste pretty good. My limp is gone and my hunger temporarily abated. Who knows? This stranger may have been intended for my blessing, a coincidental angel with the obscure soul of a saint, bringing me a gift like a rose.

PART III
LIVING AS WELL AS WE CAN

Chapter 12
FATIGUE

There's a certain slant of light
On winter afternoons
That oppresses, like the weight
Of cathedral tunes.

~Emily Dickenson

There are medical and psychological reasons for the extreme weariness that draws us like a magnet to our beds at eleven o'clock in the morning and sometimes again at three o'clock in the afternoon. Although fatigue is common in the general population, persons who suffer from systemic scleroderma and other autoimmune connective-tissue diseases seem to suffer fatigue more often and more severely. Responsibility to identify the causes falls first upon the patient or patient's family, since physicians must rely on our detailed reporting in order to know what tests to order and what interventions to recommend.

If anemia is present, a simple blood test will tell the story. Iron-poor blood may indicate an iron-poor diet, malabsorption, or more serious problem involving the working of the GI tract. In persons with systemic sclerosis, there may be a slow bleed from ulcers, polyps, or tiny blood vessels in the stomach, diagnosable by an endoscope procedure. These usually are able to be controlled or eliminated by treatment.

Various breathing issues can promote fatigue as well as indicate underlying medical conditions. Sleep apnea involves waking through the night when breathing stops for longer than normal intervals; this condition, if untreated, can damage the heart. *Pulmonary arterial hypertension* may be the cause of both breathlessness and fatigue. When cardiac output is low, dizziness and faintness may accompany feelings of fatigue. Joint and muscle pain also can rob a person of sleep, resulting in daytime fatigue. For each of these there are available pharmacological as well as natural treatments.

Depression can be a cause of fatigue. Counseling may be helpful, and, sometimes, antidepressants. People who winter in northern climates may develop seasonal affective disorder (SAD), relief from which may come with regular use of a special lamp that is a safe substitute for sunlight. Exposure to extreme cold or heat may bring on fatigue. Determining the right amount of social stimulation for one's particular personality type, extrovert or introvert, is another consideration when searching for causes. Travel, with or without careful attention to one's self-care, is also on the list.

Wherever possible, engaging in pleasurable exercise such as walking, swimming, rowing, or biking can increase available energy by improving circulation. One of the biggest losses for the person who is plagued by fatigue may be the interest in or the ability to have sex. Planning ahead with one's spouse or partner, pacing daily activities, and getting sufficient nutrition and rest, may help to foster enjoyment of intimate sharing and release.

Saturday, May 10, 2008
   I knew I'd need at least a short nap before the art exhibition tonight. Even as a young woman, I avoided after-hour events; being with large groups of people increased my fatigue. Even though I could send out a lot of sparks the first hour or so, my friends called me a party pooper.

Friday, May 16, 2008
   Seem to forget how tired I become after days of eating without thinking, and missing naps and swims. Tidied the house, did laundry, spent a couple of hours at the church office. Back home an invisible harness pulled me toward the bed. Gave in and napped for a half hour before swimming.

Wednesday, May 21, 2008

Late start. Had to push myself to prepare for the woman who does the heavy cleaning once a month. She uses the vacuum, which pulls me along like a powerful lawn mower, or a large dog who takes you down the sidewalk faster than you want to go.

Friday, May 23, 2008

Some quiet time alone every day's important. When I served as full-time pastor and lived in a parsonage next door to the church, there were many intrusions. Parishioners showed up unannounced at my kitchen door. As a servant of the Lord, I believed I was always "on call," a hard standard to relinquish, a harder one to fulfill.

Sunday, June 1, 2008

Home from the Scleroderma Walk, I went down to the pool to stretch and swim. I could easily have swum the entire mile and a half of the "Walk" around the park's pond in a couple of hours, glided along in the water without a hitch. Water is easier to move through than air, considering gravity, the hard pavement, weak muscles, aching joints, and two crooked toes. Today, I was able to walk only the shortest distance on the paved road through the park.

Friday, June 13, 2008

Memories of my youth flooded into my waking hour. Eating poorly, relationship stresses, and drinking with friends took a definite toll on my body. Later on, as a young mother, I could never keep up with the other mothers, or my co-workers. Their strength and energy always exceeded mine, or seemed to. Marriage and home life went downhill.

A physician whom I consulted during my mid-thirties thought I might have lupus, yet ordered no diagnostic tests.

He seemed annoyed that I might have an inconvenient disease. Moving to the left of the medical model, I devoted myself to reading Freud. Medicine truly fascinated me, but was impractical. I ended up going back to school to study psychology.

Thursday, June19, 2008

Fatigue caught up with me today like a little dog biting at my heels. Hardly noticed until its tiny teeth broke my skin. Definitely past time to fold up for the night.

Wednesday, June 25, 2008

The more I try to pace myself, the better. I've been reflecting today on how well my lifework has accommodated my fatigue issues. As pastor of small-to-medium congregations with no ambitions to become a bishop or denominational administrator, I was always able to fulfill my preaching and pastoral duties. Even now, as a part-time interim for a medium-sized congregation, unless caught up in an emergency situation, I'm able to nap or lie in the sunshine between three and five o'clock in the afternoon. This gives me a fresh start for the rest of the day, and a jump-start for an evening meeting.

Friday, June 27, 2008

Failed again at pacing. The good news is that I had the presence of mind to pick up take-out for supper. If I had skipped my swim this morning, the day would have played out more evenly.

Wednesday, July 2, 2008

Too tired to sit at my computer. A three-hour clinical staff meeting framed by an hour of travel each way, followed by a nap, supper, and pajamas.

Thursday, July 17, 2008

Reckless spending of my energy is catching up with me. A little while ago in my attempt to scour the kitchen counter, I dropped cleanser into an open drawer of pots and pans. My heart sank on seeing the white powder all over the cookware. I'd have to take everything out of the drawer for rinsing. A sudden wave of weakness came over me, and I decided to leave everything in the sink. I'm beating up on myself now, thinking how someone without an autoimmune disease probably would not drop the cleanser in the first place. She certainly would not walk away from a sink filled with pots and pans; she would clean up before calling it a day.

Friday, July 18, 2008

Been on my feet since 6:00 a.m., except when eating, visiting parishioners, or driving. A half-hour rest around 3:00 helped. Yet even as I lay there, the voice of my mind kept telling me: "You don't have time for this. You don't have time for this."

Then came another quieter voice, the interdiction: "Take time for this. If you don't take time for this, you won't be fit for anything else."

Thursday, July 24, 2008

Echoing of party-goers' voices late last night at our chaplain retreat combined with bursts of thunder and lightning kept me awake past midnight. I'm wrecked. The rain poured down as I wheeled my suitcase along the path to the dining hall for breakfast. Morning worship and goodbyes were a strain. Had to will myself to maintain alertness, to smile, to interact. Even while hugging and taking photos with friends, I couldn't wait for Norman, my driver, to pick me up.

Monday, July 28, 2008

Wicked tired, and it's too late to start the laundry. The only way I'll be ready for Thursday's guests is to do the wash and kitchen early tomorrow, so my cleaning person can finish up Wednesday. As for the papers and filing still haunting my desk area, I don't want to resort to hiding them in a closet.

Tuesday, July 29, 2008

I hid them in a closet. Three naps already, not all sleeping naps; just being good to myself. Up at 5:00, organized most urgent papers. Staff meeting and clients will keep me at church most of the day.

Wednesday, July 30, 2008

Once again, saved by a nap. If I can iron the tablecloth tonight, I'll be able to finish food preparation before my guests arrive in the morning.

Monday, August 4, 2008

Good results stopping work around 9:30 p.m. Making sure the lights are out by 10:15. A tame existence, but one where I can get through a day without a nap if I have to.

Friday, August 15, 2008

Dragged myself around the Bed and Breakfast most of the morning before the drive back to Nathalie's house. So tired, I fell asleep sitting upright in the passenger seat.

Tuesday, August 19, 2008

A little after 8:00 p.m. and ready for sleep. Conversation this morning with the senior pastor about a staff situation brought some peace. Glad to be home after greeting time and prayer at the community dinner. Nothing could lure me out tonight.

Saturday, September 6, 2008

Left the dinner party early so Fatigue could finish me off in the privacy of my own home.

Monday, September 15, 2008

How can I, for days, forget I require naps, wholesome food, and exercise? Why do I repeatedly fail to ask the Spirit to help me discern, to remind me to care for this body? Today I pushed myself to swim aerobically, instead staying with my usual relaxed crawl and back strokes. Could fit only three small meals into my schedule; and now, at 7:00 p.m., just beginning to wind down.

As a young mother, I would often lie on the bed to rest around 7:00 in the evening for a short nap, and sleep until morning. I know mothers get tired, awfully tired, taking care of even one child. My weariness appeared to be extreme, not only to me, but to my young son. At age eight, he produced a drawing to illustrate my malady. "The Sleeping Mother Factory" featured a row of beds on a track, a sleeping mother on each one, ready to be packed into waiting cartons and shipped out.

Hope I can stay awake for at least another hour before I'm ready for packing and shipping.

Saturday, September 20, 2008

Ate little until 5:00 p.m., because a fit of fatigue lasted all day long. This isn't scleroderma fatigue. Hours before dawn I felt a burrowing sadness, though I still can't get a handle on the reason. Had trouble doing stuff all day. The up side of leaden limbs is their affinity for rest.

Monday, October 20, 2008

So glad to see Bob waiting for me in the airport's waiting area. I began to cry as soon as we were in the car heading home. The physical and emotional toll from the last twenty-four hours added together: my fall during the touch football game in L.A.; the family's good-natured, though tiresome teasing; having to say goodbye to my grandchildren; the pre-dawn speed ride to the airport; 3,000 miles of rocketing through the lower stratosphere. The tears were a gift, actually, a relief, a little river of peace.

Saturday, November 1, 2008

So tired on this eve of reversal to Standard Time. My clocks are all turned back to tomorrow's 8:00 p.m. My body takes longer to "fall back."

Sunday, November 9, 2008

Returning home from the pastoral counselors' conference, I was tired, but unwilling to miss The Madrigal Choir rehearsal. After four hours of riding in the car, sang for another three. Exhaustion cured by close harmony.

Friday, November 14, 2008

Failed to take my half hour of lying down with eyes closed and the opportunity for all systems regulated by the unconscious to reboot.

Monday, November 17, 2008

With much too much enthusiasm, I wrote, saw clients, and shopped for fresh produce. My competence was so satisfying; I kept putting off nap time until I was weeping from fatigue. By four-thirty, the hour I'd planned to swim, had no choice but to crawl into bed.

Saturday, December 6, 2008

An athlete deserves a rest, especially a wounded athlete. Left leg and hip are still hurting from standing during our concert. Stayed home except for a trip to the grocery. Had to alternate one hour on my feet with an hour of sitting or lying-down time for rest of the day.

Sunday, December 7, 2008

Hypothermic reaction to being out in below zero wind-chill. Thought I was protected by many layers of wool and down; but the exposure brought on fatigue worse than I can recall.

Wednesday, December 10, 2008

Don't know if my tiredness is depression about my knee, the falling outdoor temperature, too many cookies, or a little of each. While resting with my leg positioned over a bag of frozen peas, I thought I'd apply warm castor oil packs to the inflamed area for several days.

Monday, January 12, 2009

After accomplishing most of my to-do list, my energy's at an all-time low. A winter with no hope of going to Florida seems longer and grayer than usual.

Tuesday, January 27, 2009

Did a little research on the Internet after getting back from my office. Napped. After supper, made phone calls, paid bills, and lay on my bed, dumbly watching a documentary about Monarch butterflies emigrating from Canada to Mexico. I watched them flying in droves past my brain. I may be still recovering from the effort of Bob's birthday event. Need to consider my limitations before planning celebrations. All week I tried to pace myself, with lots of help from my friends. There's just no way to sidestep the details of entertaining a crowd.

Wednesday, January 28, 2009

Snowbound days like this I move and think in slow motion. Fatigue lies in wait for me and, given opportunity, bounces onto my back like a soft tiger. I'm estimating the tiger's poundage as I watch the world turn white.

Friday, January 30, 2009

Three short naps without shame.

Friday, February 6, 2009

Slept well in spite of the apartment's disarray. This week I've been too tired even to pick up the mitten still in the hallway on the floor. Pieces of important tax information are scattered over the dining room table. The laundry basket overflows. As the mourning dove coos from my bird clock, I consider the difficulty of going out to see clients in the winter while trying to fulfill my commitment to self-care.

Thursday, February 12, 2009

Both body and soul incline toward fatigue. Lost more weight. Apartment's not pretty. My schedule, though lighter at the office, still requires venturing out into wind and sleet.

Wednesday, March 4, 2009

Home after esophageal procedure; am tired and ravenously hungry. Slept a while. The hospital called. The drugstore called. Bob left. There's nothing to do; nothing I want to do. Have to time the taking of my medications. After I eat, I have to stay up a couple of hours before lying down again. Lying down is my greatest pleasure.

Sunday, March 14, 2009

Sat on the couch in the living room with my feet up for hours. Closed my eyes, half asleep, hugging my knees, dreaming of a reclining chair. The scale and style of my living room couldn't accommodate even a small recliner without sacrificing needed space.

Afternoon at Barbara's. She was unusually peaceful as I'd hoped she'd be, and patient. Half reclining on a deep, feathered loveseat during our hours of reading and discussion, I nearly dozed off more than once.

Thursday, March 19, 2009

Timing my meds and eating are extraordinarily tiring. I have to fight off the feeling of digestive rebellion and remember to chew slowly. Saw one client in the morning and one in the afternoon. Sang for a couple of hours at tonight's Madrigal Choir rehearsal, always a lovely distraction and sure remedy.

Trying to finish cooking before a period of weakness hits me again is turning the kitchen into a disaster area; too tired to clean up. Even the living room, always my neatest space, has become nearly uninhabitable. I'm putting papers on the chairs and sofas, even on top the piano, instead of tossing or filing them.

Monday, March 23, 2009

My body wants to return to sweet under-the-covers warmth, which it did several times this morning.

Thursday, April 9, 2009

Maundy Thursday, several days after my second endoscope procedure, and I'm so tired. Been working at the office since early morning. Feeling guilty about missing Holy Week services, I'm listening to Handel's "Messiah" and sending up prayers for the seriously ill son of a client.

Saturday, April 19, 2009

Bob brought groceries including a chicken for soup. Been resting a lot, hoping to knock out what I think's a cold. After a little lunch, too tired to make soup. Fatigue increases when there's a drain on my system. Could the healing process be dragging me down? It seems "allergic" is a dirty word to my physicians, but have to wonder if the new drugs are getting to me.

Monday, April 20, 2009

Making a pot of soup took all my energy. What appears to be a cold is pushing me to the limit. Took some Benadryl, watched TV, and turned in early, nose sore from blowing. How can I check whether this leg-itching, persistent weakness, and congestion have anything to do with my new prescriptions, or with scleroderma?

Tuesday, April 21, 2009

Rather than preparing me for an active day, my long sleep aided by the antihistamines left me unwilling to extend myself at all. Decided to do the minimum. I wrote a list of imperatives before breakfast: "Cancel presenting at the pastor's study group; grocery shop; proof the church bulletin for Sunday." Went to bed with the sun still high in the sky.

Sunday, May 3, 2009

Feeling less fatigue in the afternoons after omitting wheat and milk products from my diet. Too soon to tell if the difference is from foods, or holding off on my meds. I should consider placebo effect also, I guess.

SELF-CARE OPTIONS

Forgive Yourself/Ask for Help

Forgive yourself for not being able to accomplish as much as you had planned or promised yourself you would. Ask for help from friends and intimates when needed. If you can afford to hire someone to do heavier cleaning, shopping, cooking, or driving from time to time, do so. You will be creating a job opportunity for someone and reserving your energy for other tasks.

The List

Make a list of every physical symptom that could be contributing to fatigue; show the list to a physician for help in identifying possible causes. Consider depression as a possibility, especially if there is a family history of depression or other mental health issues; or if there has been a recent loss at work or in a relationship.

Pacing

Prioritize the things you want to accomplish each day. Keep in touch periodically with how your body feels; do not over extend yourself. Lie down for short rests even if you are feeling fine, especially on days when you must work and/or fill responsibilities outside the home.

Schedule a daily nap if you think you might need one. Biorhythms, time, and weather changes tend to be more tiring for those with systemic diseases.

Chapter 13
WORK/LOVE

"Love and work are the cornerstones of our humanness."

~Sigmund Freud

Work and love can give rich meaning to our lives; they also can produce the greatest stress. Some persons who become physically handicapped are able to continue to work indefinitely. This usually depends on an understanding administration, supportive co-workers, and/or an individual's professional independence. Many others are not so fortunate.

Although there are several forms of love, erotic love draws couples together in committed relationships. Sexual functioning in persons with systemic sclerosis and other autoimmune connective-tissue diseases is likely, over time, to be affected by pain and decreased mobility.

There is no question systemic diseases can bring unwelcome physical changes; these changes may influence or require us to withdraw from meaningful work and relationships. In SSc, hands may curl inward from contractures and fingertips become ulcerated, sometimes requiring partial or full amputation. Eating can require a major effort. Recently, I watched a woman struggle to get food onto a fork and then slowly transfer it to the center of her narrowed mouth. Activities we've always taken for granted such as writing longhand, touch-typing, opening a jar, or walking a mile may become impossible.

The day will come when each of us is no longer able to work outside the home. For those who are relatively well maintained, this may not happen until well after the official age of retirement. For others, the day will come much sooner. Romantic or sexual love frequently takes a backseat to other needs and activities, if not abandoned altogether.

Even if you can afford to stop working and have a supportive spouse or partner, there will be a sense of loss. Most of us identify with the skills we have developed for work in the world, as well as those we use to maintain an orderly house and keep our family well and happy. So, how can we accept ourselves when we can no longer hold a pencil or lift a cup? Would we be able to buy a voice-activated computer and work at home? What if our financial resources fail? If a person is alone and financially strapped, should she, or he, make arrangements to share living quarters with a friend a relative? These are questions that we ought to ask, and solve if we can, soon after diagnosis.

In the middle of consuming health issues, who among us is going to worry about having a love life? Couples who experience a decrease in or discontinuance of intercourse because of joint or muscle pain do not usually go for counseling. They imagine there is no solution. They may stop their affectionate touching, as well, because of hand impairment or embarrassment. The falling off of sexual expression may cause additional stress, guilt, and complicate the identity issues of both individuals.

There are many with disabling conditions who have not given in or given up. I've been inspired by persons who struggle to find new ways of engaging in work they love, and new ways of making love with their spouses or partners when the old ways are no longer possible. For more than a year I have watched couples in the scleroderma support group meetings. Often the husband or significant other has become a part- or full-time caretaker; yet the two retain the aura of lovers. I have watched them smile at one another, touch, and make affectionate remarks. I recall, also, reading encouraging stories in *The Scleroderma Voice,* a publication sent quarterly to members of the Scleroderma Foundation, about individuals who continue courageously to confront the most difficult of medical challenges: the sort of story in which a pianist, for instance, with contracted fingers might begin composing music; or a teacher, unable to continue classroom teaching, becomes a writer of children's books; or a nurse becomes a volunteer telephone operator within her hospital's health services department.

My dear friend Bro lived fourteen years with a heart transplant. He encouraged me to call him Bro; and surely was like my own brother, calling and staying in touch even when we couldn't get together. He continued his financial consultant business by communicating with his clients via computer, working when he had the strength. Although he enjoyed work and a loving extended family, and had friends all over the country, he had no spouse or partner to share his gift of time.

Many couples avoid discussing sexual intimacy issues. This is unfortunate because such conversation, while difficult, can open the door to renewed pleasures. A loving lover can always find ways to embrace, to kiss, to be tender with a spouse or partner even when hands cannot grasp and muscles and joints fail to move as once they did.

Meaningful work and intimate sharing are the highest forms of adult play. This is good reason to persevere in both as long as we are able. Having to relinquish work or intimacy represents a tremendous letdown. If we can see our specific limitations as challenges, we may we be able to find more hopeful solutions; however, this is not always possible.

Until I turned fifty, leading a congregation was more fun than anything I could imagine, being together with a community of people who loved me and whom I loved. Now, as pastoral counselor and spiritual director, my joy is more inward, an honoring of others' trust, an invitation to become a partner in bringing about longed-for transformation in a client's goals or relationships.

Learning to write for publication doesn't stop me from dreaming about painting watercolor portraits. Our weekly art class has a few students with hands severely bent from arthritis, yet each is able to convey her way of seeing color, space, light, and line. One student who has studied art with a famous artist and teacher continues to create beautiful work. Being able to communicate one's unique way of seeing the world is not as dependent upon the condition of our hands as on the clarity of our vision.

The following journal notes involve my work and recent retirement as a church pastor, as well as the slowing down of my pastoral counseling practice. For the sake of personal discretion, I have withheld my history of intimate relationships.

Thursday, May 8, 2008

I'm not sure writing in this journal every day counts as work.

For about a year, I've been employed one-third time as an interim pastor, side by side with a Presbyterian minister; we share preaching and pastoral care. This qualifies as work, yet is often surprisingly creative and freeing. We are temporary leaders in a cathedral-style church going through hard times, a situation common to many churches these days. Every two weeks, I write a new sermon. I never stop editing and rewriting until a few hours before delivery. At the moment of truth, I really don't want to consult my script. I want to speak without notes, which sometimes I do.

Thursday, May 15, 2008

Took communion today with a woman who is remarkably matter of fact about dying. "Dying is boring," she said, "I would like it to be over." She talked of not being able to do the things she'd like to do; she spoke of wishing to have a pet, a dog or a cat for company when family members are working, and for nights when she's alone in the house. There's no one to walk a dog during the day; and she knows her days are numbered.

Something sacred about breaking the Bread of Heaven with a dying person. I hoped she would feel closer to God; and prayed she'd experience, even in the hard part of leaving earth, something more interesting than dying. In her last weeks, the woman's family arranged for her to stay with them and their pets at their country house from which she made a peaceful and reportedly good-humored exit.

Monday, May 19, 2008

Must make a radical change of pace if I'm to keep working. Hours juggling church and counseling responsibilities keep me from things I ought to be doing for myself. Don't have enough energy for everything. My Albany rheumatologist says people with diseases like SSc ought to steer clear of caretaking roles. After today, I think he might be right. Every person who came to see me, cried. White birds flying out of the tissue box, one by one. I kept thinking of these lines by William Blake: "Can I see another's woe, and not be in sorrow, too." Sounds like a question, but it's really a statement.

"No, Mr. Blake; I cannot," was my mind's rejoinder.

Tuesday, May 20, 2008

Drove early to the hospital to be with a woman scheduled for same-day surgery. To avoid creating a disturbance in the small waiting room, I held her hand and whispered the prayer right into her ear.

Wednesday, May 21, 2008

Enjoyed the hour's drive to the meetings my counseling colleagues convene.

Except for our clinical director, each of us is pastor of a church, part- or full-time. Our clients are referred primarily by churches and former clients. At monthly meetings, we spend the first of three hours sketching the high and low points of our lives and practices. After briefly going over any business issues, we are open for case presentations. Each of us, except our clinical director, has an assigned supervisor for individual monthly consults.

Friday, May 30, 2008

Visited two parishioners in their nineties, each bright, well-read, and in touch with the world. Conversation, prayer, a glass of water, and affectionate banter makes a fine afternoon. They inspire me to grow as old as I can.

Monday, June 16, 2008

Anxious about what will be decided tonight at the meeting of church leaders. Will I be asked to sign a new contract? Will I be preaching only once a month until November or December when things will change again? On one hand, I'd like the cut off to be sooner rather than later. On the other, I'm sad this may signal my practical retirement as an acting pastor.

Sunday, June 22, 2008

Lots to do on a preaching morning. Bob listened to my new ending on the phone at 7:30 a.m. Hungry and exhausted after the service, too tired to eat, I crawled into bed before noon and happily lost consciousness. A late lunch, and time in the sun with my paperwork. Seems all I do is work, eat, exercise, and sleep. Family time with Bob and hanging out on the co-op patio is all that keeps me in the stream of ordinary life.

Tuesday, July 1, 2008

Went back to church to greet the guests at the weekly community dinner. Tonight there were around eighty. Some bring their families. Almost all are poor, living on the edge. There are stories of alcohol and drug abuse, malnutrition, and chronic illnesses. I say hello and offer my hand, which is grabbed or held, shook or kissed. A touch can break barriers. I recognize many of these people by now and know their names.

Volunteers in the kitchen begin work in the morning, preparing the food. During the meal, servers listen to individuals' concerns from their posts. There are many hugs. I'm always humbled by the affection I receive and ashamed of the skimpy amount I give. My job is easier than working in the kitchen. Two men run the electric dishwasher for more than an hour; they wash and put away the plates. We have real dishes and flatware, no paper plates, no plastic cutlery. Even

the cups are pottery or glass, a sign of hospitality in a world
of throw-away things.

Friday, July 11, 2008

A funny day. Ideal, really, because there was nowhere I
had to go. Time to dream. Later in the day brought an example
of how a dream can be dangerous. A long-distance coaching
client considering a job off the beaten path is thinking of
leaving his solid profession to interview for what he considers
his dream job, an art and entertainment form that may be
short-lived. I ask about the broader intentions for his life. I
remind him he's in his sixties, divorced, and carrying a load of
debt. I'm tempted to say certainly he has the option to explore
this new opportunity. Instead, I keep my mouth shut. At last,
I quietly reinforce the conservative option: staying sane and
centered and not running away with the circus.

Was I wrong? Sometimes I want to run away with the
circus.

Thursday, July 17, 2008

A beautiful drive to my supervisor's. We focused on my
few clients who came initially seeking short-term, solution-
oriented counseling, but did not terminate after meeting their
goals. Instead, they continue to schedule monthly visits.
Wondering if I ought to be firm about ending contracts. My
supervisor suggested they may be using me as a touchstone in
their life journeys.

After reviewing cases, I told him about my identical
dreams from last month, how he and I had greeted a parade of
unearthly humans. During the telling, I began to realize how
he has been a touchstone person in my life journey. Priest,
spiritual director, and guide, he's the male reflection of who I
am and am becoming.

Friday, July 18, 2008

Two parishioners in the nursing home were doing poorly and grateful for a visit. The woman had been wheeled early to the dining room where she sat slumped over in a wheelchair. She brightened at my greeting and said, "I love you." The man, bedridden, was weaker than a month ago; though, his hand, when I held it, was warm and alive, not so much the hand of a seriously ill old man as a bird or other small creature with a beating heart.

Saturday, July 26, 2008

Last night I worked too close to bedtime. Paid a pile of bills, shopped, went to the bank. At 10:00 a.m. talked with my son who probably won't be able to complete his house project before his family returns at the end of the week. Like me, he seems to work all the time, loving it, mostly. Just hope he's not unconsciously imitating his mother's compulsive style. On retreat this week, I was the black beast of the work ethic. Silently, I judged the presenter who did not work hard enough for my taste.

Saturday, August 2, 2008

The next sermon may be my last for a while: "Dreamer, Take Heart." The dreamers I have in mind are not only Old Testament Joseph and New Testament Peter from today's readings. The other dreamers are the senior pastor and me. He's worked hard to encourage this congregation to consider merging with other churches. The practical goal is to eliminate the cost of maintaining three cathedral-style sanctuaries. The spiritual goal is to insure these dwindling congregations will have the resources to continue to reach out to the poor in our community over the next twenty years. Trying to shift the focus from preserving a beautiful sanctuary to preserving the lives of people in need isn't easy. We understand their reluctance. The chancel of the church in which we serve features a large Tiffany mosaic of Jesus as a boy in the temple; the columns are trimmed with gold leaf. Our pipe organ is the one professionals play on when they come to perform in this city. The music directors and soloists are opera singers. The pews have comfortable cushions. The real Jesus, who prefers the poor and marginal people of the world, may seem an unpopular task-maker.

Back to my message: Sometimes dreamers, like Joseph, get thrown into pits by their brothers. Peter, another biblical dreamers, thinks he can walk on water, but hasn't enough faith at the critical moment to succeed at overcoming surface tension. No matter. The best thing about God's dreamers is that they never give up, even when they are banished, sold to the Egyptians, even crucified. Nothing, not even death, can stop them.

Monday, August 4, 2008

The answer was in my email. The senior pastor has given notice of his resignation, which means I go, too. I'm saddened, and exhilarated.

Friday, August 9, 2008

Enjoyed conducting a wedding for a bride who is within a few weeks of her due date. Although the ceremony was last-minute, the marriage has been intended for a long time. Was impressed by the family's avoidance of excess, their emphasis, on the couple's act of commitment. They decorated a private dining room at a local restaurant with modest bouquets, set up an acceptable altar by covering a table with a white cloth. I brought a standing brass cross from church for the temporary altar. After the service, we had a sit-down dinner in the same room. All in all, a sane celebration.

Finished "Dreamer" message; may have to update in the

morning. Some concern about my co-pastor's resignation letter being read just before my sermon. Hope the congregation's reaction to his leaving and my meanings will mesh somehow. I don't think most of them realize this terminates my contract as well.

Sunday, August 10, 2008

My sermon delivery was airborne. "I love the recklessness of faith; first, you leap, then you grow wings." (William Sloane Coffin, 1924-2006) Even Bob, who put up with listening to portions on the telephone, said: "You hit a home run!"

Tuesday, August 19, 2008

About an hour ago, drafted my goodbye letter to the congregation. I'd like to be able to keep my counseling office in the same building, stay in the background. No more pressure to write and print sermons or visit parishioners on bone-chilling days; just pay my rent and see my clients.

Friday, August 22, 2008

Started making goodbye visits to homebound parishioners and those in nursing homes. I was more prepared for their sadness than mine.

Friday, August 29, 2008

Got to the nursing home an hour earlier than scheduled with no reason I can think of for being early. As I was leaving the unit, I recognized a woman in the parking lot, a member of a church where I once served as interim pastor. The family was gathered in the sick room around her mother, and she was anxious that their pastor may arrive "too late." She accepted my offer to be with them a while.

The sound of the dying woman's labored breathing dominated the room where I sat in the circle of family members. We talked quietly for a while until everyone stood together for prayer. I put one hand on the sick woman's head and the other in the hand next to mine. I sat with them again until conversation waned.

This unscheduled visit gave me confidence to break with my long-time employment as a church minister. I realized today I can serve where I am at the moment. God will get me there, whether by whale, like Jonah, or by Toyota.

Monday, September 2, 2008

Our church staff gathered for a goodbye lunch. I ate my vinegary salad slow as a snail. Clearly, this was end time for our ministry here, and for mine perhaps anywhere, at least formally. The parting hug with my co-pastor was a comfort.

Tuesday, September 3, 2008

Much on my to-do list is related to one job instead of two. I'm attempting to separate myself from the hub of church activity while working in the same building. My rented office at the end of a long hallway is a little closer to China than the main office, which may be enough of a boundary.

Wednesday, September 24, 2008

Put in a couple of hours trying to increase my client load. With the economic downturn, fewer people can afford a skilled listener.

Thursday, October 2, 2008

Surprised how relaxed we were tonight, he and I, soul friends from the beginning. We talked little. He rubbed my back while I sat in a chair. Then I rubbed his back. We might have been married once and forever in this lifetime if the planets and our souls had been in the right alignment. This relationship shifted my reality more than any other.

The strength of the bond amazes me, how our love, though not fulfilled in a sexual sense, seemed to have begun a long time ago. In a book about reincarnation, I read about souls returning to earth becoming involved again and again with the souls who were important in their former lives.

Friday, October 24, 2008

Woke up at 4:30 a.m., nervous about today's interview for a church position. By midafternoon, I had become a most unwilling candidate, but felt caught in a dilemma of obligation. I would never have sought this out; they called me. Back home after the interview, I felt sad, and tired to the bone. I lay down on my bed. Instead of taking a nap, called my friend Nathalie. She reminded me how stressed I used to get whenever I had a list of parish visits to complete before the end of the month. She was right. Within the hour, I called the interviewer and withdrew as a candidate. Immediately after making the call, I relaxed, revived. Getting off the hook unhooked me from a heavy weight.

Friday, November 21, 2008

Woke with a dream of being in my mother's house still fresh in my mind; I'd asked her if I could move back into our old house that my brother sold long ago, now inhabited by strangers.

This dream fits my category of unconscious gold. Tatters of yesterday seem to have gone into its making. Last night before sleep, I listened to a concert on public television by two violinists, violinists like my mother. Earlier in the day I was working with a client who is trying to differentiate from her mother; easier said than done.

I have to consider whether, like my mother, I have chosen a life of all work and no play, even though my work has nearly always involved creativity and pleasure. When my mother was not yet fifty, an attractive widow, she shut down her personal needs and became entirely devoted to teaching and performing. Although I knew of more than one man who wanted to date her, she stayed determinedly single. For several years, she played viola in the state orchestra. On learning the auditions for violinists were closed; she learned to play viola, tried out, and was accepted. I was both proud of her musical achievements and sorry for what she might have missed in a later-life intimate relationship.

Tuesday, December 2, 2008

This morning, a lovely dream. The man from my soul life was sitting at a table, shirt sleeves rolled up as they would be in summer. I walked over to him and stroked his arm. I've always loved his arms.

He said, "I miss holding you."

I said, "Thank you for saying that, because lately I doubt."

I did not have time to think any more about the dream, which gave sweetness to a day of steady productivity.

Wednesday, December 3, 2008

I'm tired as a grizzly pulled out from her hibernation burrow. With so much to do before the weekend, I was awake at 3:00 a.m., on the computer by four, working until after five on my end-of-year report, then back to sleep for a couple of hours. Not liking the night shift. Nevertheless, enjoyed the drive over the country roads to the staff meeting; miles of snow-covered branches against a blue sky. My colleagues helped me make a decision about a client I'm evaluating. They were right; she is more appropriate for a clinic setting. Too much mystery about her diagnosis and previous treatment.

Driving back, sailing into a pale sunset, I struggled to keep my eyes open and stay alert.

Tuesday, December 23, 2008

Soul partner called, and showed up. We ate lunch, talked for about an hour. Before he left, he helped straighten out the Oriental rug, which hasn't lain flat since the window installers were here. Those were our best moments, on our knees behind the green couch pulling together on the gold rug. Over the years we've not had many chances to pull together. He mentioned he'd like to avoid eating when he comes by because it takes time away from conversation. This, after devouring every bite of the ample lunch I'd prepared. What's wrong with him? Eating is ordinary, everyday life. If there is no everyday life for him, there never could be an everyday life for us. In the hallway, I watched him put on his coat and shoes. We embraced before he disappeared. His lips were like a feather across my cheek. Unfathomable man.

Tuesday, February 17, 2009

All my clients were tuned into their respective issues. One, a woman near my age, remarked at how relaxed I seemed today. When rested and relaxed, I know I'm more present for my clients. State of being may be as important as any verbal feedback I can give them.

Tuesday, March 10, 2009

Enjoyed my afternoon clients, all women over fifty. With most women, relationships are paramount: husbands, children, grandchildren, ex-husbands, boyfriends, and for one, God. When they learn to care for themselves, they draw back a little from their emotional involvements. They claim their solitude, their joy, their spiritual paths, each with its own dynamic.

Tuesday, April 7, 2009

Certain clients remind me of the way I persist in taking

on too much. My youngest is under more pressure than she's willing to acknowledge. I'm trying to ask her the right questions, trying to coax her into awareness. Sometimes I wonder at how much listening to my clients teaches me.

Saturday, April 25, 2009

Held a graveside service for the mother of two sisters; each traveled a long distance to be here. We watched the cemetery official lower the urn into the little square grave. The sisters threw in their lilies and roses, one by one. There were three of us meditating death on this hot, sunshiny, spring day. When they cried, I cried. We had to wipe our eyes with our hands. A pack of tissues would have been welcome, and bottles of cold water. In the eighty-five-degree noonday heat, we had neither.

Sunday, April 26, 2009

Scheduled to be guest preacher at my old church, I was awake at 2:00 a.m., trying to think of an ending for my sermon. As I lay there, the words began to come to me through the darkness, the way they came to prophets of old or, in this case, to an old prophet. I turned on the light to write them down. Worked around the apartment before going back to sleep at 4:00.

Preached with more spontaneity today than if I'd had to produce a printed version. No windsurfing this morning, no flight, just a thoughtful meditation about the sense of loss for the first disciples, and for us.

SELF-CARE OPTIONS

Job issues

Part-time work may be better than full-time for people dealing with serious health issues. If other household members can carry the financial load, scaling down spending may be wiser than for the patient to continue the pressures of full-time employment. This solution may be a necessity for mothers with scleroderma who are parenting school-aged children.

Psychological Issues

Those who identify strongly with their work have a harder time postponing or ending career involvements. Even a temporary break for treatment can feel as demoralizing as permanent retirement. Having a trusted confidante, counselor, pastor, or close friend with whom to talk over feelings before, during, and after termination, or transition, can be a great help.

Although adults who swap work and childcare roles may find the arrangement difficult at first, successful adjustment is possible. When a swap has been made so the parent with SSc is able to stay closer to home, everyone can benefit. Children have the opportunity to develop a new closeness with the parent who was accustomed to working all day; and the spouse who was staying home, or working part-time, knows that by working full-time, he or she helping to balance the family's home life.

Relationship Issues

There are many forms of love to nourish us and those we care for; all forms require commitment. In couple relationships, preserving tenderness and passion requires diligent practice and, occasionally, consultation with a marriage or family counselor. Love for our family, our friends and neighbors, our community, and love for the farthest places and people our hearts can reach expands the gestalt of our healing network. Love, in time, becomes our "work."

Chapter 14
TRAVEL

"Life is either a daring adventure or nothing at all."

~Helen Keller

The word travel brings up images of faraway places. For people with systemic sclerosis even a trip to the grocery store on an extremely cold or sweltering day takes planning. The health issues we deal with at home do not disappear when we are away from home, and they span the continuum. Most common of these: reaction to temperature changes, digestive problems, fatigue, and muscle and joint pain. For many, circulatory issues and/or breathing difficulties are also on the list.

A certain amount of anxiety accompanies the prospect of travel for almost everyone, particularly if one must travel alone. When taking a plane trip, for instance, assistance must be arranged in advance for in-airport transportation, oxygen tanks, boarding, and other details.

There are ways of keeping pace with the trips that fit our regular work schedules, and visiting patterns. Taking time to prepare for predictable needs can make the briefest sojourn safer and easier. Equipping our cars with bottled water and extra clothing, enlisting a friend or hiring a driver for trips longer than our energy bank can afford, and mailing non-perishable diet foods that cannot be carried on a plane are a few ways to smooth the adventure. Such preparations, while time-consuming, offer the best opportunity for a pleasurable journey.

No matter how carefully we prepare, hours waiting in an airport will be tiring. Change in altitude is another unavoidable aspect of air travel. Rail travel varies widely in degrees of comfort; even newer trains may rock and rumble on old tracks. A cruise on a quiet river can cause seasickness; and being a backseat driver in one's own car, with a hired driver, can produce an anxiety attack in the hypervigilant. Nevertheless, the prospect of getting out of the house for a couple of hours, or days can lift one's spirits. Where medically feasible, planning trips to see family, friends, or favorite places is usually worth the effort.

> Thursday, July 24, 2008
> Returning from a week at the chaplains' retreat, sorted mail into piles for prioritized opening. Emptied my suitcase right away, so don't have to face it tomorrow. Oh, to lie in my own bed again! To stretch into sleep like a drowsy feline.

Cross-country Weekend: Getting There

The plane to Detroit took off in the rain before sunrise. I prefer smaller planes, including turbo jets with loud propellers. Low tech has the appeal of simplicity. After turning the reading lights off, I could see a cushion of navy-blue clouds beneath us. As the clouds thinned, the lights of towns appeared. The first half hour, I had to work hard trying to stay warm. Gathering my jacket closer, I tried to huddle deeper into a seat colder than the surrounding air. When I drummed up courage to ask for a blanket, the steward gave me two. At last, warmed and relaxed, I sank into silent prayer for the flight, the passengers, and our respective journeys.

In a while, my thoughts were flying ahead of the little plane. When I see *that* former husband after more than a decade, will I be able to give him the late apology that I promised myself at the Yom Kippur service? The last time we met was in Woodstock years ago. We carried the birthday cake and presents up to the second floor to celebrate his father's ninety-fifth birthday and our granddaughter's first. His father was an artist. Some of his oil paintings, portraits and landscapes, hung in our apartment when our son was small. Lately, the old man had been mostly confined to bed, cared for by round-the-clock household companions. Our grandchild, just learning to walk, spent the party hour clinging to the furniture handles of a dresser, struggling to stay upright.

As I exited the plane, an attendant was waiting for me. After a call on her pager, she took off immediately, promising to return after answering a summons to another gate. After falling in this airport a few years ago while running to catch the tram, I was advised to travel "handicapped." Stranded in the wheelchair, I waited for ten minutes. The airport temperature must have been between fifty and sixty degrees. Although wearing a wool cap, gloves, and scarf, I saw no advantage to freezing in place. I wrote a note to the attendant, which I placed on the seat of the wheelchair, informing her that I was on my own.

I tried to maintain an even gait as I walked through the long corridors, up elevators, into the tram, and through the tunnel of psychedelic colors moving against a sea of painted clouds. Exhilarated by my independence, I rode the speed-walks. When wheeled through this tunnel last year, self-consciousness blocked my awareness of surrounding sights and sounds.

Since my scheduled layover was about four hours, I inquired about World Club, which is a pricey way for passengers to endure a long airport wait. The advertisement tempted me; the Club offered snacks, spring water, and computer access. I longed for a chance to put up my feet, a deep leather chair in which a nap may be possible, a computer to email my son; and I was hungry and thirsty. My packed lunch, however, would not be welcome there. On the way to my gate, I noticed from the flight display that another plane on my airline was scheduled to leave for L.A. in one hour. An official I encountered suggested I sign up for standby.

If the ability to walk through the terminal was the first sign of good fortune, the second was conversation with Gail, a psychologist also on her way to L.A. to attend a meditation retreat. We spoke of vicissitudes of the soul while I devoured my egg salad sandwich. Our visit also distanced me from my anxiety about whether or not there would be room on the earlier flight, which eventual certainty was the third sign of the day's good fortune.

I was assigned the least-favored middle seat; but my neighbors kept their bodies closely wrapped in sleep, permitting me to use the armrests on both sides. At every opportunity, including when my seatmates roused themselves to go to the john, I did arm pushups against the baggage door, and discrete leg bends. I drank lots of bottled spring water and tea, and ate my fruit and cheese.

After landing, I pulled my small carry-on to the shuttle pick-up and called my son to announce my arrival. An hour later, I was comfortably ensconced in my hotel room, opening the windows and peeling off the bedspread.

Thursday, October 16, 2008

For our granddaughter's birthday dinner, Nomo [my husband before Bob] treated us to a sushi bar, where tempting selections traveled around a great oblong track. Seated next to the track, we helped ourselves to tiny color-coded plates of freshly made sea-based creations. As we dug into smoked eel delicacies, I told the grandchildren how my grandmother caught live eels in the Shark River inlet near her summer house in Belmar, New Jersey; how she cooked them on her old coal stove; how good they tasted even without the gingery sauce and spices—the sort of story where kids say yuck and adults stare expressionless at their plates.

Friday, October 17, 2008

Like a summer morning. My son worked on the kitchen cabinets in his open-air workshop while Nomo and I sat on the deck, talking about church work and finances. He is a lay leader who teaches church school and volunteers at their weekly soup kitchen. Driving back to the hotel, I made my long-deferred apology for being a runaway wife so many years ago. He was gracious, admitting that marriage had not been his specialty, either.

This evening began on a stressful note. My son's exasperation at his son's incessant teasing of his sister led to an angry reprimand with a swat, uncharacteristic for a parent who never spanked his kids. Our grandson lost his balance, falling on the concrete floor of the parking garage. Presenting a skinned elbow to document his outrage, he began to scream. Everyone needed time to cool down. I suppressed my desire to be peacemaker. Letting them work this out together was the way to go.

My son's family took off in two directions while Nomo and I went into the restaurant to wait for their return. The emotional uproar resulted in a later meal; but, at our reconvening, the children were soon talking and laughing together, the boy leaning affectionately on his father's arm.

For most people, handling relationship issues during family visits is as tiring as travel itself. When the visits are infrequent, there may be effort on all sides to fill every shared moment. The inevitable let down comes in a day or two. Children get cranky. Hosts grow weary. Guests begin to long for home.

Over the past ten years of making these cross-country weekend trips, booking a hotel room has proven to be well worth the cost. A quiet early morning, an afternoon nap; breakfast and, sometimes, lunch, are under my control and an antidote to jetlag.

When a friend exclaims: "You're going all that way for a 'long weekend'?" I answer, "Yes," with a smile.

Saturday, October 18, 2008

Watched the cabinet-making proceed in the sunny backyard workshop until, at my grandson's request, I went to his room to help with his school history project. He dictated from his bed, sitting among his paper notes, while I happily keyed in and edited.

We spent the afternoon at a large mall. Nomo had the wisdom to avoid this junket by hiding out in his hotel room. Malls to me represent a kind of torture unrelated to occasional joint pain. I'm worn out by the dizzying multiplication of objects, colors, and smells. The trudging through furniture and toy stores was sweetened only by being with the kids. By lunchtime, we were all irritable.

Tonight, we sat around the table in their pretty little house enjoying vegetables in curry over rice.

Sunday, October 19, 2008

Unremarkable morning. While the kids were at church, Nomo and I purchased food to sustain us through the next day of air travel. All afternoon, everyone sat around the house, reading the newspaper or wandering into the backyard. By three o'clock the kids were asking to go to the park to play touch football. I demurred. They begged so charmingly, so persistently, that I gave in. Nomo, a big man, made a lurch to avoid being tagged, accidentally knocking me over backwards. I landed on hip and head. Saved by California's spongy grass and my woolen visor cap. No bleeding, just a little headache and stiffness in neck and shoulder. My ever-compassionate son grabbed my cell phone to photograph me lying on the ground. The photo's still in the inbox to remind me how easily "touch" can turn into "tackle."

A few years back, basketball laid me low. My grandson was teaching me how to make a basket: jump and shoot. There's a photo of the two of us, airborne, him guarding as I made my thrilling way to a basket. I limped for three weeks.

The evening's home entertainment featured a spoof my son wrote caricaturing our relationship. My head still aching from my fall, I withdrew into poorly concealed gloom. Goodbyes were next. Hugs and endearments swallowed up my last ounce of energy.

Monday, October 20, 2008

Nomo took me on a hair-raising ride to the airport in the pre-dawn. Caught up in the current of speeding traffic, we missed the sign for the car-rental. Darting from lane to lane, looking for a U-turn or alternate approach, cars and trucks speeding by, at last I spied the turn to airport and car rental.

Wednesday, February 4, 2009

A cold morning. I packed up spring water, greens for the salad, and cooked rice for lunch at Bob's; he'll buy the fish. His house is on my route. I also made guacamole for the staff meeting as a way to avoid sugar and salt snacks.

Drove over hills, beautiful under a layer of clean snow. Warm and well fed, I sang along with my Taize CD. I dream of going Taize, a mission community in France whose musicians compose, lead the singing, and accompany their beautiful harmonious chants. At staff meeting, we began by telling our recent adventures. I described Bob's birthday knighting, and passed around a photo of him standing at the front of the chapel with his deer-in-the-headlights expression the moment he realized the party was for him. Three hours went by fast; case presentations kept things moving. Driving back, I watched the winter sky grow darker. No matter how carefully I try to protect myself, meeting days in winter wear me to the bone.

Saturday, April 11, 2009

Devoted all morning of a fourteen-hour day to my third cousin's birthday party near the city. There is no way I could have got there without a driver. Delivered from negotiating heavy traffic and navigating unfamiliar neighborhoods. Norman simply programmed his GPS. I sat in the backseat and looked out the window.

Norman's an easy guy to be with; we've developed a structure for our day trips. We stop for a break about every hour and a half. We each take along personal supplies, spring water, and snacks. Today we left early enough to visit my brother and sister-in-law on the way. Their house is right off Route 80. Norman hung around out back, in and around my car, a happy camper, eating lunch and listening to his books on tape while I visited with family.

Sitting comfortably in my brother and sister-in-law's living room, I downed my protein drink while two beagles panted at my feet, had some rare conversation with my grown nephews re: their career and girlfriend interests. My brother and I made jokes about our aches and pains; he has arthritis. My sister-in-law and I caught up on family news. Filled a few glass bottles of water from their natural spring source and gratefully received two pounds of ground venison, which I secured in a well-insulated portable cooler. Changed into my white wool suit just before leaving for the last leg of the journey.

The rest of our daylight driving, my time was taken up with writing the "few words" and blessing I'd been invited to give at the birthday event. I wrote, rewrote and edited, committed to memory, and practiced in my mind so I could be fully present to the company of guests.

Seeing my relatives was mostly a treat. Also met and conversed with more than a few interesting strangers. We sat in assigned tables of eight. To reach the microphone, I had to walk the length of the long dining room; I straightened my posture as much as I could. Guests laughed at my opening quip in response to my second cousin's introductory remarks—her saying that my father was a wild guy, someone you would not expect to have a minister daughter.

I countered, "He wasn't just a wild guy. My father was the playboy of the Western World!"

Took my pills and ate the banquet food with neither appetite nor interest. No reflection on country club's chef; my GI tract's still rebelling. Norman brought the car around at 8:00 p.m. to spirit me away. Leaned on my pillow in the backseat for many miles, reviewing the day with pleasure; was delivered home before Cinderella midnight. Glimpsing my image in the hallway mirror, I didn't look much the worse for wear. The white wool suit was beginning to bulk under my storm coat. Home, thank God, is about taking it all off.

Wednesday, May 7, 2008

After a night of intermittent wakefulness, I left for my appointment in Albany with friend Barbara at the wheel. Hadn't taken my proton-pump inhibitor (PPI) because I didn't feel like eating at 5:00 a.m. I'm supposed to eat half hour after the pill. Hadn't seen Barbara in quite a while, so we were talking too much, too early.

SELF-CARE OPTIONS

Car

Keep a first-aid kit containing standard antiseptic and bandage-making items, including sample amounts of medications. A cooler comes in handy for foods and/or medications requiring refrigeration. When away for more than a day or two, take a blood-pressure cuff if used regularly at home.

Glass or stainless steel bottles with glass linings are better than plastic for carrying filtered or fresh spring water. These materials will not leak toxins when the temperature rises.

A blanket, extra jacket, hat and gloves, and hand warmers in the car summer and winter could help with the surprise of temperature changes both in and out of doors. If you are exposed to cold air conditioning, or your hosts prefer a cooler environment, backup warmth is readily available.

Train

Trains permit personal food items not served or available for purchase onboard. Extra packages may require a porter for help with transport to and from the sitting/sleeping area. On long-distance train rides, ice is available to refill a cooler. Insulin is safe and portable when kept at a low temperature.

I've taken overnight trains from New York to Chicago, from New York to Fort Lauderdale, and from Los Angeles to New York. For some, trains provide a relaxing alternative to plane travel; one must like the sound of wheels clicking along the tracks, the constant motion, and be able to endure unexpected delays.

For those with dietary concerns, Amtrak serves basic fish and chicken entrees every night. For vegetarian options, you may have to call ahead. I found the vegetarian dishes on the regular menu too spicy. Their green salads were excellent and served with little packets of dressing on which the ingredients are printed. After I had just begun to follow a gluten-free, cow-dairy-free diet, I fared rather well traveling cross country by train.

Plane

Buying insurance at the time of purchasing airline tickets is wise. Should a traveler become ill before or during the trip, fare or rebooking fee can be reimbursed. Acceptable documentation of illness or accident is required.

If traveling "handicapped," schedule extra time between flights because of the possibility of delays. Having to wait for a wheelchair or electric cart can cost time and stress.

A word of caution about traveling "handicapped": Unless standing or walking is dangerous or problematic, consider leaving a "borrowed" wheelchair in order to board the plane later with the other passengers. Boarding early may be a problem for those with lung sensitivity, as some airlines use air fresheners between flights. This was once a problem for me. The smell is strongest before most passengers begin boarding. Allergies to products, chemically similar to scented candles and popular home air freshener sprays, may require wearing a filtering mask, available from any pharmacy. If a passenger is coughing or appears ill, a mask over nose and mouth may protect against contracting another's illness. Air circulation on planes means "what goes around comes around." Using a saline spray before a plane trip and/or lining the inside of one's nostrils with a thin coating of petroleum jelly may help. Hand sanitizer can be used to clean hands, sanitize the food tray; and even wipe the bathroom seat.

When sitting for long periods, there is the danger of blood clots forming in the legs. Support or compression hose may help. Get up at least once an hour An aisle seat frees one to stand, stretch, or walk more frequently than a window or center seat. When a passenger in a nearby seat gets up, it is possible to do modest stretching exercises. When trying this, stay aware so as not to block the aisle for other passengers or airline personnel.

Packing food for air travel may be smarter than chancing a selection from the flight menu. A see-through container of fresh fruit, nuts, salad, and cheese is easy to get past security and can last all day. Bottled spring water is freely distributed by flight attendants as are other non-alcoholic beverages. Hydration is important while flying, and helps to keep all body systems in balance.

Travel light. Smart packing is a science. For those who prefer not to wait at baggage claim, a modest wheeled carry-on and large fabric handbag can hold clothing and accessories for a week. There is usually someone willing to lift them in and out of overhead compartments.

Hotels

Take off the bedspreads; they are not washed often and may be dusty, which could interfere with breathing. Extra blankets in the room or those available from housekeeping will be cleaner and just as warm. Try to get a room with a window that opens. Avoid using combined heat and air conditioning units, even for ventilation; they almost always have mold in the filters. Hand sanitizer is good for cleaning the telephone receiver and TV remote. These may be rarely cleaned and may carry the germs of previous guests.

For those who sleep on a bed raised several inches to discourage GERD, telephone books or magazines can be placed underneath the mattress.

Chapter 15
OCCASIONS

"I am not in this world to live up to other people's expectations,
nor do I feel that the world must live up to mine."

~Fritz Perls, psychotherapist, author (1893-1970)

When we are feeling well, holidays and other special occasions can bring delight and meaning. When we are feeling unwell, they may seem to make cruel demands for our last drop of energy. Taking the time to evaluate where we are on the health continuum, physically and psychologically, may help smooth the path to more enjoyable participation in celebrative events.

Holidays can become exhausting when the primary focus is on special foods and gift giving. Depression may be the result for people who entertain unrealistic expectations of joy or fulfillment. Physical limitations compound the stress for those with fixed ideas about what a holiday requires of them. Aiming for simplicity in both preparations and gifting is wise.

The old adage, "It is better to give than to receive," may be true; but for many of us receiving is harder to do. Close friends and relations usually understand when people with scleroderma have periods of weakness, fatigue, or pain, and want to be helpful to us. If we who are living with the disease are too concerned with keeping up our image as a "giver," we may miss out on the many gifts, visible and invisible, coming our way.

One question we may have: "How can we enjoy the pleasure of receiving when we feel we have so little to give?"

On Mother's Day in churches where I've served, I've directed the children walk up and down the aisles, presenting every woman in the congregation with a flower, whether she was a mother, or not. The pleasure children take in giving is the whole lesson. The joy of a true giver is innocent, wanting only reassurance the gift is received with joy.

Birthdays and anniversaries are traditionally happy times. They mark the occasions of our growing and our loving. There are years when these may turn awkward, even painful. Those sadder birthdays and anniversaries, the ones reminding us of the loss of someone dear, are unavoidable. Grieving for a lost job or a pet also is common and deserves respectful acknowledgment. Individuals with systemic scleroderma have told me they have spent a year or more grieving for *themselves*, for the persons they used to be before their diagnosis.

During periods of mourning, we may put aside social and other occasions for a while. However, to continue to avoid friends or family celebrations can be as detrimental to our health as the disease itself. Our mortal package requires enduring periods of sadness and grief from time to time. However, if we are serious about caring for ourselves and our intimates; we must do all we can to reconnect with those around us, to welcome times of relaxation where we are likely to laugh more and to worry less.

Where death is neither premature nor tragic, there is always some laughter before, during, and after a funeral or memorial service. Sorrow at a loved one's passing goes hand in hand with celebrating a life well lived, which includes humor and happy memories. After a religious service of beauty and authenticity, the shared food, the stories, and the family "reunion" are intended to begin the healing of the loss.

Stress tends to increase with the size and complexity of the occasion. Wedding and other large parties may be the worst. We may feel pressure to dress a certain way; to buy a gift that we cannot afford or to travel a great distance. The host of such an event may or may not have control over how things transpire. As an invited guest with a close relationship to the bride or groom, unless you are able to document being under the knife at precisely the time of the event, there may seem to be no acceptable excuse. As a member of the wedding, you have a keen sense of obligation. This can make canceling out extremely difficult.

Preparing friends and relatives in advance for the possibility of having to cancel at the last minute for health reasons is a good idea. For those times when you are feeling too ill to leave home and must send your regrets, there will be less regret because others have been warned about the possibility of your canceling.

Unrealistic expectations of ourselves or others can ruin any day. At important gatherings, expectation-lowering may protect one from disappointment and even enhance the event. Large gatherings, especially with family, may increase the stress on some of the guests and on the hosts. The hosts may not be able to meet everyone's expectations, needs, or their tastes. Sometimes I cannot find one thing on the buffet table that I can eat. Often, I will contribute a favorite dish of mine, and others can share.

As I perfected the discipline of expecting less from others, I began to have more fun. When anxiety diminishes, creativity is free to roam. We don't have to talk simply to fill the silence. Remarking about something in this magnificent universe that deeply attracts our interest is the best way to prompt discussion, and the old rule about focusing on others rather than ourselves still works. Demonstrating the hospitality we desire to receive is the surest method for having a good time anywhere and almost always requires our moving outside the boundaries of expectation.

Friday, May 30, 2008

Tried to get a tricycle for the Scleroderma Walk next Sunday and found out there's not enough time for Joe to borrow one from another store. I'll have to see how far I can go on foot.

Saturday, May 31, 2008

Before eating, we remembered in prayer those who gave, and are giving, their lives for our country. When I was a child, we had no cookouts, no marinated meats on Memorial Day. We stood on the grass at the cemetery in the sunshine, watching a float covered with flags and flowers wind slowly down on the river while a trumpeter played taps. Those occasions were

part of something sad that made me weep, that made me want
to heal the world.

Friday, June 6, 2008

Usually I fly cross country for my son's and grandson's
birthdays during the first week of June; this year I stayed
here for the Scleroderma Walk. I was thinking this morning
about my son growing up, how beautiful he was at seven—at
seventeen, how smart. While I love and admire the man he's
become, I still miss when he was small. I could hold him and
touch his hair. My grandson's still at an age where he can be
held. I miss him, too.

Friday, July 4, 2008

A good day for weeding out papers, swimming, and
sunning. The family cookout was fun. I wore my faded, red
T-shirt with the blue star at the center. Maybe we ought to
progress in this country from celebrating Independence Day
to "Interdependence Day." Peaceful coexistence may be hard
for most to imagine and harder for political leaders and a
people schooled in war to attain. I know it takes guts trying to
be a peacemaker, even in my own family.

Fireworks, on the other hand, require no work at all; I
have only to pull aside the curtains and look up. When I first
moved here, I'd get up out of chair or bed to watch them,
amazed at my easy access to the colorful sparks exploding.
After a year, I waited until the finale to make my move, when
the bursts become louder and more frequent. Now I listen to
the crackling and the cheers from under the covers, sometimes
falling asleep before the finale.

Wednesday, August 13, 2008

Nathalie and I are sitting on the sundeck of one of those
houses on the ocean, our feet up on the railing, watching the

boats on the water and sunbathers packing up to go home. There are hundreds of old Victorian houses here; my favorites are the ones with lacy cutouts painted in odd pastels with flowers growing everywhere, hanging from porch ceilings and spilling out of big pots on the steps.

Thursday, August 14, 2008

Nath's still sleeping. I've been up a couple of hours doing everything I can to make this a good day, starting with my yoga stretches on the floor of the sundeck. Sat here for almost an hour, writing a poem for tonight's reunion dinner:

Like an ancestral clan,
the seagulls are gathered on the sand, watching the sunrise.
Kayaks, smooth as loons, glide beyond the sea's ripples.
Runners and bikers open the beach;
dogs are walking their owners.
I'm up early to catch the first drop of ocean air.

Tonight we'll miss the dear ones
too frail to gather like gulls this year.
We'll lift our glasses in a toast to them
before we dig into fish and pasta.

Anticipating flight, we, like gulls,
with gliding wings and side-view eyes,
will laugh that we are still alive; and here
to celebrate our centurion, Marie
who is winning the Olympics of longevity
in this intimate competition for wine and love.

Sunday, September 14, 2008

Today received a beautiful send-off from the church, a huge party cake, thanking me for "years of love and care." Though sad to leave, was able to celebrate without regret.

Thursday, November 27, 2008

This year my brother and sister-in-law invited me to go with them to visit her parents on Thanksgiving. While I'd love to be with them, the long drives to and from these destinations hold me back. I am thankful for everything, for my body's systems working as well as they are, and for a relaxed afternoon with Bob and family.

Thursday, December 25, 2008

Wheeled a pushcart brimming with presents through the hallway, down the elevator and to my car before 9:00 a.m., promising myself I'll purchase all gift certificates next year. Most of the presents were for Bob's family tucked into gift bags with colorful tissue paper frothing out the tops. Stuff for the children wrapped and bowed because gift bags don't offer the fun of bright paper torn off in handfuls and scattered on the carpet.

Christmas with my son, his family, and other relatives ended years ago. We cheer by phone. Here, a new family has grown on rocky upstate New York soil. I put the roast in the oven at Bob's house and the presents under his tree. I arrived at the neighborhood Lutheran service shortly after 10:00. The sung liturgy, the carols, and the Bread of Heaven are what I wanted most this morning: "The gifts of God for the people of God."

Rest of the day, preparing the table, cooking, and watching glittering packages turn into ordinary pajamas, games, and books. When conversation waned, I came home, went straight to bed so I could go back for the evening feast with the late arrivals. No responsibilities this time, just greetings and a piece of sugar-free pumpkin pie.

Walking into my apartment door was the most wonderful moment, getting under the covers of my bed, hot water bottle against my feet, beyond compare. Merry.

Saturday, February 14, 2009

Just returned from the grocery store when the security guard called from the front desk, saying I had a package. I saw a vase of red roses as I stepped out of the elevator. For years, I've admired bouquets of flowers on the shelf in front of the elevators; but they've always been for other residents, never for me. This time, my name was on one side of the card. On the other: "Happy Valentine's Day from Your Knight."

Wednesday, March 4, 2009

March 4th is the day my father died. When we were married, Bob and I used to go to Florida all of March. I'd wake to the sound of the mourning dove and start walking up Ocean Avenue toward the Catholic church to acknowledge my father's importance in my life. None of us know the location of his ashes. My stepmother took the urn after the funeral lunch and, since then, has been out of touch with all of us.

On those March mornings in South Florida, I'd walk about a mile along shore before or after Mass. I put a fresh rose in a small vase beneath the statue of Mary, or else lit a votive candle that would burn for a week. Since my father came from the Roman tradition, as did his mother and the aunt who raised him after his mother died, and since they were devoted to St. Francis of Assisi, I figure he's a Catholic whether he went to Mass or not. Although apparently lacking a sense of religious identity, my father remarked to my uncle on the night of my ordination: "Now we have our priest."

Walking back to the seaside rental those March days, I breathed more easily, comforted by my small memorial. Thoughts of my father kept surfacing today, with no opportunity to make a gesture of remembrance. All morning, I was in surgery for my endoscope procedure.

Sunday, April 12, 2009

Easter. No part of this holiday was easy, but the church's decorations themselves provided a powerful proclamation about resurrection. A huge paper maché stone had to be moved away from the door of the sanctuary before members of the congregation could enter. New life flowed from the movement of hundreds of colored streamers hanging in the nave. They danced in the morning light.

Our family meal was good although we had a protracted discussion about sibling strife.

The sad postscript to this Easter Sunday came months later: news of Bro's death. Most people referred to him as "Newheart," his email handle. His sister and I agreed by phone, if he had to die, Easter Sunday was the right day. Bro is the man who had been resurrected from his own dead body after what appeared to be an unsuccessful heart transplant. He told me the story a dozen years ago when we were the only two persons in the pool at a small resort in Lauderdale, how they unplugged the life-support machines when the transplanted heart failed to beat. Incredibly, his situation spontaneously reversed. His new heart began to beat, and all systems were "go."

Shortly before Easter, Bro decided to sign out of the hospital. He wanted to die at home by the Jersey shore where the sea breeze has a briefest journey from surf to bay. Nathalie and I spent a week in his downstairs apartment one summer. I picture him sunning in a lawn chair until the moment he was taken; he never worried enough about his skin cancer to stay out of the sun. Our main concern had always been those seventeen immune-suppressant drugs he had to take every morning, all sizes and shapes, many-colored, almost as beautiful as the sea-glass he collected in jars.

Another cancer killed him, nothing to do with his heart. The afternoon I spoke with his sister, part of me wanted to continue in relationship with his family, and part of me shied away. There was nothing anyone else could add to our story. Bro and I were the ideal brother and sister, all friendship and trust and laughter. Only wish I had the chance to say goodbye.

Thursday, May 7, 2009,

Carried out last May's intention to have my driver take me to see my Albany specialist. I'm looking forward to relaxing in the backseat on the way there and back. After a hard year medically, there may be possibilities for continued improvement, especially around changes in diet and exercise. I'm hoping my specialist will have some new ideas or information about my recent health concerns. I bet he'll laugh when he reads this, and tell me to lower my expectations of him!

Chapter 16
STRESS

"There is more to life than increasing its speed."

~Mohandas K. Gandhi

Negative stress exemplifies our at-oddness with ourselves and with the world. Stress shows up when we magnify our regrets about yesterday or our fears about tomorrow, is frequently accompanied by pains of one kind or another, and believed to be a contributor to disease. In fact, the wrong sort of stress is such an obvious factor in progressive illnesses that there is usually no reference in medical indexes, including those about scleroderma. Physicians in the research and writing fields are understandably focused on more specific manifestations of their disease specialty.

Interestingly, there are not only references to stress in two books by patients with SSc; there are thought-provoking discussions. Karen Gottsman's *The First Year—Scleroderma* (Marlow & Company, New York, 2003) in "Month 10" entitled: "Living: Stress and Your Disease," devotes a few pages to avoiding stress whenever possible. Mark Flapan's book, *Perspectives on Living with Scleroderma,* contains four short essays on the theme, "Why Suffer Emotionally More than Necessary?" His writings have been enriched by the many persons he has known with scleroderma, some of whom he met while leading support groups. His objective was to help others to cope with the predictable fallout from living with a rare condition and, sometimes, the expectation of a shortened life.

Having struggled ourselves with bouts of stress and anxiety may help us to recognize its dangers. Certainly, after the shock of diagnosis has passed, just knowing we have a serious disease produces ongoing concern. For many of us, hurried patterns of living and working have been the rule and even may have become part of our personalities. Few realize how the fast track can affect our bodies' systems. Our hearts may beat faster or erratically, our blood pressures spike, and our heads begin to ache. We may find ourselves awake too often at four a.m.

There are psychological predilections for stress, a stringent work ethic, for instance. Sadly, workaholics are often regarded as more important than others in society. Complaints about being stressed may be interpreted as a kind of boasting to build up the false "better" self. Sometimes the workaholic begins to see herself/himself as a special person expecting special treatment by others, even after the stressors are removed.

Here is some unconscious gold from my past. While a seminary student, I was serving as a part-time pastor to make ends meet. I worked hard in my courses and with my congregation. One night, in a dream, "God" directed me to take not only the week of vacation I had planned, but two-weeks, presumably as a reward for my hard work. "God" expressed further approval by giving me a new name: "Reverend Responsible."

I woke up laughing. Since then, I have thought often about this dream, usually when I'm feeling pressured and imagining the work assigned me is more important than anything else.

Here is my fresh interpretation of God's directive: "You're doing okay; don't knock yourself out."

I have a nine-by-eleven-and-a-half-inch book calendar with tasks written in for most hours throughout the day. The year I buy a smaller calendar will mark a real turning point. Committing to pleasurable, relaxing times is easier for me when a challenging activity is involved, such as learning new music, or being taught how to draw a human eye. Even when I swim with my pool friends, I try to limit casual conversation.

"You're here to swim," my mind keeps telling me, or "You're here to practice deep leg bends." Freud would note an overactive superego.

Recovering from our compulsions takes effort. When life's highlights have been mostly work challenges, a person's worst times will probably be periods of sickness or inactivity. No matter what we do, or don't do, anxiety about our perceived identity perseveres. Here are some questions I ask myself with others you may be asking yourself:

Who would I be if I could not work outside my home?

Who would I be if I were not able to do all the things I've always done, such as caring for my family, for example?

How will I feel if I give up not just one, but both of my professional involvements?

How would I feel if I joined a support group and began to draw closer to other persons with scleroderma, some of them considerably handicapped?

Will I still be who I am if I have no project to complete? Could I be content hanging out with my friends in the building, or spending a few afternoons a week with my sketch pad?

Will you still be you, will I still be me, if there are unwanted alterations in our appearance?

SSc can slow us down to the point where our mobility is severely limited. To resist changing our familiar habits is natural. The inner changes we must make can be more difficult than the external ones. Work less and relax more? Spend forty minutes a day in exercise and, perhaps, additional time, even hours each day, involved in other self-care practices? Lean a little more on friends and family? For me, every one of these is easier said than done.

I've begun canceling clients and meetings when feeling unwell. I used to bite the bullet and push on. When the temperature drops below twenty degrees, I avoid going out. I'm more able to accept help when offered. I passed up an attractive preaching invitation recently which, a few years ago, I would have accepted. I've begun to practice saying "no." I have gone from regarding stress as unavoidable, to an entirely different mindset. I am becoming receptive to a new way of being, and of being with those I love.

Although anecdotes on the subject of stress can be found throughout the journal entries, the ones I've chosen for this chapter will, I hope, encourage readers to consider taking a lighter approach to living in a world that presents not only unpredictable medical challenges but unpredictable joys. May we always to be able to welcome the unpredictable joys.

Wednesday, May 14, 2008

Disturbed by the fluctuations on Wall Street, called my financial advisor about transferring my modest mutual funds into a money market. He admitted the year's decline shook him, too, and didn't try to deter me. He brought the papers for signing right to my office. I was surprised by his respect for my decision since he's the expert. Getting stressed about money's a bummer.

Saturday, May 17, 2008

Entertaining at home is avoidable stress.

Sunday, May 25, 2008

Beginning to understand the desperation of people living with systemic sclerosis. I've been at the brink of desperation myself more than once. If I were worried about becoming a fatality any time soon, I might be running down every treatment I could find, no matter how unusual or untested.

Scleroderma is an "orphan disease," a term that makes me reminisce about my early life. I had two living parents. I was not an orphan. However, stress was written into my script before the word came into vogue. Around the age of four, when my mother was ill, the paternal side boarded me for a year in a convent orphanage.

I'd always attributed my physical symptoms to early-life trauma; psychologists call it somatic conversion. There is no question I had stored old grief in my body: gut, lungs, muscles, and bones. Where I got into trouble was assuming my symptoms were unique, and could not be diagnosed.

Tuesday, June 3, 2008

Made more progress with finances. Decided to pay off my car loan while I'm still working more than half-time. The eight-percent interest I'm paying out is a lot more than

I could earn by investing. I've noticed when I'm anxious about something, I aspirate more than usual. Well, I've done everything I can to get the money problems out of the way. The coughing and throat-clearing isn't going away, so must be something else.

Tuesday, June 17, 2008

Felt sluggish all day, no energy, worrying about losing my church job, I guess. The threat of recession's shaking everyone up, particularly retired people who've been using investment income for paying bills. Omitting undue stress, whether for love or money, is my summer goal. Just signed up for a July learning retreat offered to United Methodist chaplains and pastoral counselors with the theme: "Care of Body and Soul." Trusting the leader will take on the subject of stress.

Sunday, June 22, 2008

Need to buy food; make salad dressing, shop, visit the nursing home, and get to Bob's by six. Happy my next scheduled sermon is not until August. Home and hospital visiting are lighter responsibilities. Although I've been preaching for decades, there's still something daunting about standing before a crowd of people who have come out on a sunny summer morning to hear a word of hope.

Thursday, July 17, 2008

Planned to hand wash and wax my car at Bob's. I keep a hose, soaps and sponges in his garage. He tells me I'm crazy to wash the car myself. I've persisted because the Toyota dealer warned that commercial car wash services can ruin chassis and paint. The temperature outside was already ninety degrees, so I decided to take Bob's advice and try the old-fashioned car wash in his neighborhood, with no frame to bend the chassis. I drove right onto the concrete floor where the sprays are. The attendant skillfully wielded a big, soft brush; and I saved myself a huge hassle at half the cost of the automatic wash.

Wednesday, July 23, 2998

Ongoing stress does damage to all body systems. The causes may be complex, but the lesson is clear. For starters: avoid corn syrup, inactivity, and toxic people at home and abroad.

Saturday, August 2, 2008

I've been noticing some people at church distancing from me. This may signal the end of our ministry before the end of the year.

Saturday, August 16, 2008

If only I could put tape over Roberto's mouth! He's such a reliably excellent cook; I shouldn't criticize his out-of-kitchen behavior. He does not talk; he raves. His negative monologues about politics, religion, food, and the economy are predictable rants. I've learned to go upstairs after his gourmet feasts to quiet down before sleep. Let the others stay at the table; I'm just a houseguest protecting my peace. He is the sort of long-time friend we are commanded to love as family, in spite of his social abrasiveness.

Saturday, August 23, 2008

A line from my goodbye letter to the church: "I credit my co-pastor and his cows for improving my sense of humor both in and out of the pulpit." His lifelong avocation has been working on a cattle farm; his sermons often highlight comparisons between human and cow psychology, usually brilliantly funny and with full allegiance to the faith.

Wednesday, September 17, 2008

Needed more sleep than I got, ate some chocolate and other delicious bad stuff to relax. Warning: chocolate may be an antidote to stress, but has big bad side effects!

In the wake of hurricanes in the Gulf of Mexico, now the near crash on Wall Street. My first impulse was to withdraw money from my savings, to hide. After some thought, realized mattress banks can be as hazardous as the Federal Reserve. Glad I unloaded those mutual funds; but what about my long-term care insurance?

I've always had had an exaggerated urge to prepare for possible emergencies. Collected lots of bottled water and non-perishables before the millennium, the winter Bob and I rented a studio apartment at the Florida shore. All of January and most of February, we drank the gallons of bottled water. Soon grew tired of Cheerios and canned tuna. Odds and ends of the surplus traveled back to New York with us on the auto-train.

The peaceful millennium did not wholly put to rest my fears about national emergencies. The media still touts the wisdom of having a week's supply of food and water in our homes. Today, as many days, I've had to dig into my "week's supply."

I have friends who won't deal with troubling possibilities, the ostrich strategy. They tell me they've stopped reading or listening to the news. To me, this choice conveys isolation, not a stress-free solution. Until the day that we're offered convincing proof of friendly inhabitants from other galaxies, this planet is all we've got. I may be one individual in a globe-full of humans, but human is the community to which I belong and must somehow learn to negotiate.

Tuesday, November 11, 2008

Too much effort getting the place shipshape for a visit from my soulmate anti-hero. Cleaned off the dust the window installers left on the piano and tables, ate four good mini meals, dressed in my best casual clothes, and waited. When he didn't call by 7:00, I called to ask if he was coming over.

Thus has it always been. No return call. He's lost among the stars. Fell asleep early, trying not to care.

Wednesday, November 12, 2008

Cried a little this morning over last night's disappointment, but determined to make this the best of days. Free until nearly 3:30 p.m., I worked out for a half hour. Nathalie and I had a marathon telephone conversation. I asked her to try to make me laugh. We laughed over her failed efforts to do this on demand.

Thursday, November 20, 2008

Was hungry when I shopped, hungry when I got home. Ate too fast, too late. No triathlon today, no pool. Cranky, I'm blaming this on poor planning. I'm a colossal time-management failure. A few phone calls took two hours. My late-afternoon client continued to talk ten minutes after I had begun making moves toward the door. Attending to each detail today seemed to take an eternity.

How hard it is to change my behavior, to overcome the urge to do everything but take care of myself.

Wednesday, December 24, 2008

Stayed home tonight, remembering Christmases past, serving my first churches, where idealism and zeal kept me on a steady treadmill for God. Never much of an administrator, my offices were rarely presentable. I poured myself into preaching and pastoral care, with the excuse that these were my gifts. For each of the seven years after leaving seminary, I came down with laryngitis immediately after the Christmas Eve services. I'd sing the descant to "O Come All Ye Faithful" and, as the midnight chimes rang in Jesus' birth, my voice completely disappeared. Before bed I'd be gargling salt water, happy as a clam. For the next ten days I'd do nothing but make tasty soups, sleep and, when I got my voice back, talk on the phone with my friends.

Not until writing my paper for clinical-pastoral education did I realize I was planning these stress-related sicknesses as surely as I was planning services for the Nativity. Even after I was able to interrupt the pattern, I wondered sometimes if my best vacations may have been those winter weeks in my little parsonage on the Delaware River. Whole days to watch the falling snow and write Christmas cards before the deadline of Epiphany on January sixth.

Monday, December 29, 2008

I woke at 4:00 a.m. with anxiety about things I cannot leave to chance. Turned on the light, ate some cottage cheese and crackers, too hungry to wait until daybreak. Made a general priority list and a list for today. I intend to avoid social involvements until January, and to move more intentionally into my spiritual life, work on this journal, and organize my apartment. Last but not least, I'd like to tame my paper plethora for the New Year.

Thursday, January 1, 2009

The photo for the month of January on my new Drew calendar got me down. Don't like the way the pillars of Mead Hall reach up into the night. Because of the surrounding darkness, they seem a sad illustration of what is left on earth when our time is gone.

I remember a January trip to Israel, pressing my palms

against the 2,000-year-old pillars in Capernaum, feeling the smooth stone warmed by the sun, stone once part of the synagogue in which Jesus is said to have preached. After returning to my church in New Jersey, I dreamed night after night about pressing my hands against that warm limestone. Midwinter longings require a brighter image than snow-cold pillars against a night sky.

Wednesday, January 14, 2009

An incident today renewed my childhood fear of monsters under the bed. Having arrived at Bob's, I'd braked in his driveway when, all of a sudden, the automatic garage door opened part way. This was shocking because Bob's car was not in the garage and, if he wasn't home, who was operating the garage door? First thought was that Bob, having seen my car pull up, may be in the house, pressing the button near the kitchen door. Guessed his car was in the repair shop.

All of a sudden, the garage door opened fully, yet still no clue as to the operator. If Bob, he'd be standing just inside the kitchen door, leaning out, waving me in. Usually, I can see the light coming through that door. Not today. If he knew I was parked outside for several minutes without entering, he'd have come out to see why. Hide and seek is not his kind of game.

I began to get suspicious. Maybe Bob was out driving his car, and an intruder had entered the house. Unless the intruder was armed and waiting for his victim, why all the opening and closing of the garage door? I pulled out onto the street and called Bob's home number. No answer. I called his cell phone. No answer. As soon as I put my foot on the gas to drive away, the garage door began to close again. Too spooked to hang around any longer.

Drove around the neighborhood, thinking of calling the police. All the while, could not help but notice I had no visceral feeling of fear, no signs of stress anywhere in my body. While imagining a dangerous individual waiting to entrap me, I felt strangely relaxed.

Blocks from the house, I got a call from Bob, saying he was late leaving a grocery store and would be right home, I told him about the garage door and suspected intruder.

"Probably some electrical thing," he said.

We arrived at his house simultaneously. He went inside to check all the rooms. I remained locked in my car and promised to call 911 if he didn't come out in two minutes. He returned to say the coast was clear and told me to park my car inside the garage. After I parked, he pressed the button near the kitchen to close the garage door, which closed on cue. Then, as I made a move to get out of my car, the garage door, which was now behind me, began to open.

"See, it's doing it again!" I shouted.

Bob came down the steps and peered into my car. He asked if the lost remote might be somewhere inside. Nice to have a logical friend. We searched various compartments and looked under the seats. When I lifted the pillow supporting my lower-back, eureka! My rear end had been controlling the garage door. When I moved forward in seat, the door lifted a little. When I moved back to put my foot on the gas, the door closed.

This story may have fable power. There are certainly psychological implications. For instance, a lot of negative stress comes from the way we think about things. Many people experience anxiety when there's no objective threat. There are also those able to deny the presence of danger, but I don't think I'm one of them. It helps me to confer with a friend about a mystifying situation such as deciding whether or not to call the police or the doctor.

Tuesday, February 10, 2009

Since work has been central in my life, identifying as retired seems a scary prospect, as though termination from the workforce implies termination of the life force. I might get more comfortable with the idea if I could see what will take its place.

Thursday, February 12, 2009

Felt pressed for time at the health food store this afternoon. A nutritionist was teaching customers how to make little rice pancakes from a brown rice batter. Hungry, I ate two of them. At the same time I was eating, I was talking with the cook, and bobbing back and forth in the aisle around my shopping cart, trying to see if there were items on a nearby shelf I wanted to buy.

Another customer at the pancake-making table instructed me to: "Sit down," and "Chew slowly"—what I need to remember to do when nobody is watching.

Saturday, March 21, 2009

The subject of stress came up again today in conversation with my friend Marianne, an RN with lupus. She said even a slight upset at work or in her church community can decrease her stamina so severely she may need to rest at home the following day. We discussed the distinction between self-care and babying ourselves. We agree that playing the sick role, acting in a way that demands special attention or deference, is not something either of us wants to do; although the temptation can be great. Husbands and even children, after a setback in their wife's/mother's health, often settle into the role of caretakers.

I asked Marianne if, when she was a child, there was anyone in her household who played the sick role, someone from whom she may have learned the behavior.

"No," she said, "I learned by myself," and explained how she went through a difficult period after the onset of her symptoms. Becoming more and more dependent on her husband and daughters to take over the responsibilities of driving, shopping, cooking, and cleaning, she had given up more activities than she believed were necessary. As she become stronger and adjusted to her drug therapies, she took back her household tasks. She values her involvements as administrative nurse, church musician, and wife and mother more than anything she might gain from playing the sick role.

I told Marianne I learned the sick role from my mother who had poorly maintained insulin-dependent diabetes for almost forty years. Widowed shortly before I left home, my mother lived with my younger sister and much-younger brother in our childhood home. After their emancipation, she lived in the house alone. With the onset of her blindness, she could no longer teach violin and piano, and moved to a residential home. At first she was angry at losing her independence. In time, however, she came to relish being cared for at the residence. Until her final weeks, when she succumbed to renal failure, she remarked about the luxury of having attendants bring her meals on a tray, and snacks to her room.

My mother lived out the example of a sick role, which gradually transformed into a positive acceptance of her very difficult medical situation. At the end, her contentment came from genuine thankfulness for being cared for by a loving staff, and her faith's assurance she had nothing to fear in leaving earth.

Tuesday, April 14, 2009

Can't seem to get started today. Almost lunchtime, and every room has exceeded the limit of chaos. Desperate for a quiet place, where phones don't ring, where there's no kitchen duty, I spent an hour this morning, reserving five days at a monastery later this month. Sometimes I've found miracles in places of peace.

Sunday, May 3, 2009

What I am savoring now is being home, with no sheep or monks or bells, in my own dear bed.

SELF-CARE OPTIONS

• Consider seeking professional help to solve financial problems, even extensive scaling down of your lifestyle.

• Try to become more aware of eating too fast, or gobbling up fats and sweets when feeling stressed.

• Use restraint when planning events, way before your calendar looks too full.

• Continue to laugh, play, exchange ideas with family, colleagues, and trusted friends.

• Tell your sorrows to a compassionate listener; don't hide them away too long.

• Eat, sleep, and exercise as though the basics matter, because they do.

Chapter 17

SPIRIT

"I have come closer to God during this illness; my faith is strong.
I wake up every morning and say thank you for another day."

~Anonymous

I was moved to hear these words from a woman who is severely disabled from diffuse scleroderma. There are others like her, people I have met or heard about, who continue to proclaim God's goodness even when their lives are a continuing struggle to eat or to breathe.

When I was a nineteen year-old university student, a professor told the class we were too smart to believe in God. I bought his view, temporarily, until I was forced by illness to look again. Making a case for belief in the transcendent/imminent is not an easy task. Most of us accept the way of seeing the world through our senses. Seeing the world through the lens of reason, as in philosophy and mathematics, also provokes little resistance in most people. Spirituality, on the other hand, especially within the structure of a religious system, is often disregarded or denigrated as a form of unreality.

In the beginning chapter of Kyriacos C. Markides' book, *The Mountain of Silence* (An Image Book, Doubleday, 2002), the author gives credence to the construct of three realities: The eye of science and the eye of reason are joined by the eye of contemplation. The third reality issues from the discipline of systematic spiritual practice. Brought up in the Greek Orthodox tradition, author Markides, a sociologist, became an agnostic while studying at university. Logic led him to abandon his faith until he became involved in a research project about monastic life. The research as well as the mentoring he received from monks with whom he worked called him back to his spiritual center. An important part of Markides' story is his observation of the evident healing powers of monks he came to know during his study project.

I have spent my life believing in and trying to speak about a God of Love in Christ. To be honest, there is a way, an intellectual way, in which I know nothing. There is another way, however, a deeper way, in which I am certain that a Heart of Love greater than any of us can imagine is caring for us every minute of every day and, not just for you and me, but for each creature on this and any other habitable planet.

I cannot answer the questions about why so many children and younger adults die of illnesses, or are taken by war and other tragedies. In matters of faith, experience is paramount. "You have to be there," as the saying goes; and still, we cannot fully understand. Even Jesus' first disciples had a hard time interpreting these events.

For anyone courageous enough to take stock of his or her spiritual walk, childhood memories may be the place to begin. Were you held, loved, cherished by one or both of your parents or caregivers? I hope so. Was at least one of them a member of a community of faith, active in reaching out to others and wholesome in its teaching? Was your mother, father, or parent substitute able to demonstrate steadiness and courage when confronted with life's difficulties? Did you grow up belonging to a religious community where you were happy to be present, where you made friends and discovered that you had talents worthy to contribute? I ask these questions to acknowledge the imperfectness of most people's faith histories. Every walk, as every leaf, has its own design.

The memory of being forced as a child to attend religious services has kept some away from adult involvement. If this is your story, you may be willing to search for a community where your heart and imagination can be fully engaged. Simply realizing you have a choice can be liberating. As there are healthy and unhealthy ways of approaching diet and exercise, there are healthy and unhealthy ways of religious thinking and practice. There is wisdom in avoiding groups with no active mission focus and no regulating administrative body, as these may turn out to be cultish and try to control their members.

If you were abused in any way by a religious official, pain and anger may deter reconnection. Pastoral counselors and spiritual directors are trained to help with the healing these wounds. Moreover, enlisting a trusted companion to lead you closer to your spiritual center may open you to new understanding of your life purpose.

Growing spiritually presents challenges. Learning to live more fully in the present is one of them. We may pray for more strength, but we are wise to be thankful for the strength we have. As people with scleroderma, if we are not already partially or wholly dependent upon another or others for our care, the day may come. Maintaining a gracious attitude as the recipient of care may be more important than the attitude of our caregivers. Being able to accept help in a cheerful and relaxed manner can mean the world to your companion.

I have known professional caregivers who for years have daily assisted chronically ill persons in their homes. These caregivers sometimes become closer to their patients than the patient's own family. Their charge may be very ill and very old, yet the caregiver has tended to this individual as tenderly as she would her own child. I have seen these women, and home caregivers are usually women, attend the funerals of their patients. They grieve as those who have known and loved the one they cared for, because they did.

When a religious institution names mission among its list of service commitments, it may be referring to helping Third World countries or to helping people in a region of our own country who have suffered a catastrophic event. Medicine, education, rebuilding, and farming are common areas of assistance. Photographic documentaries may be shown to congregations to bring members closer to the reality of a particular community's existing needs. This is where writing a check can be meaningful. When, as a group, we witness a peoples' need, we often can do much more than as individuals trying to decide how, why, or where to contribute. Mission does not always happen at a distance; mission can be local and immediate. Serving meals to neighborhood people who are hungry or lonely, and offering clothing and pantry supplies, are common local missions.

The truth is: we may prefer being givers to being receivers. Those of us with chronic diseases may someday be the recipients of others' helping hands. Here is where our built-in resistance to appearing weak or dependent certainly can get in the way of spiritual growth. When people tell me about not wanting to be dependent, I agree with them about how difficult dependency feels, how unfamiliar. If there is an opening, I also tell them the healthiest dependency is dependency on God.

Try to consider a person's offering of assistance as a sign of the Spirit's intention. This includes the ministrations of friend, partner, spouse, or neighbor. Our loved one's "mission" may be to help us through the practical struggles of living with a debilitating disease. Our "mission" may be to gracefully receive a loved one's help, realizing we would do the same if the situation were reversed.

Perhaps we can receive the gift of faith most completely by experiencing God's love in our lives. My experience, maybe yours as well, includes having witnessed the unexpected healing of someone who was given a hopeless diagnosis. Did the new medication save him or did prayerful intervention, or both? Then, after his healing, another question, an important one: To what purpose will he use his new life and healing? The goal of all healing and restored function, according to Edgar Cayce and the practice of true religion, is service to others.

However we call upon Goodness, every person must follow his or her own spiritual path. There is no way to piggyback on another's process. My journaling began as a way to motivate others to become more aware of both the value and challenges of self-care; my journaling ended up motivating me. If, indeed a cure becomes available for scleroderma, or for anyone's present disease entity, we will each continue to live in a place of existential unknowing, although perhaps more easily than we do now.

In the majority of cases the hoped-for miracle doesn't happen. I cannot describe well enough the impact of watching a person die with grace. Prayer, love, presence, and peace—these are essentials of the invisible realm. I believe we are here to learn them as well as we can and to teach others their blessings.

Thursday, May 8, 2008
    I couldn't get out of bed this morning or any morning if
    I didn't send up a prayer for the things I'm scheduled to do;
    the things I'm not scheduled to do, but probably will; and the
    things I will never get to.

Tuesday, May 13, 2008

Lying in the dark, reviewing my day, sinking into wonder about the universe, I'm thankful Aunt Betty came through this morning's hip replacement surgery. There were concerns about her heart function and general frailty.

Wednesday, May 14, Wednesday

Drove an hour through lovely countryside to have dinner with long-time friends, Max and Geri. Max and I were pastors in New Jersey when his Parkinson's was first diagnosed. A man of remarkable strength, his creativity and perseverance would be impossible without his faith. Since his medical retirement, he's written two books. In the second, *Grit and Grace*, he tells about serving churches in Paterson, New Jersey, during the civil rights movement in the 1960s. He and his wife loved and protected the people of the Black community in the face of racial anger and destruction.

We enjoyed delicious food, caught up on family news, including photos. I made them laugh with inventive recounting of my interim parish work.

Tuesday, May 20, 2008

What about the suffering in the world? What about personal suffering? Where is God in all this? Who is God in all this? What is my responsibility toward suffering neighbors? No human being can sidestep pain and grief. Why do some people get so much more than others? I wish the God whom I call Love would help me sort this out.

Saturday, June 29, 2008

Watched the orthodox Jewish families dressed in their Sabbath clothes walking to their synagogue on my street. While living in the Washington Heights neighborhood of New York City, we got to know an orthodox Jewish family in our co-op. They walked up a big hill to temple every Friday night and Saturday morning. David, the father, was a theology professor, and Carol, the mother and my close friend, was a graduate student in sociology. Carol and I, both tall and slender, were so similar in looks and mannerisms that people in our building thought we were sisters. Aaron and Rivkah played almost every day with my little boy. I saw in them a healthy example of "doers of the law."

Here, in this much smaller city's co-op, I have Jewish friends who regard orthodoxy as a trap, a narrow-minded system that promotes ignorance through insularity, an insularity that can blind its people even to their own history. I agree; there are definite drawbacks to strong fundamentalist leanings in all religious systems. Certainly this has been and continues to be true in Christianity and Islam. I am suspicious of any belief system that makes a point of excluding or diminishing those who believe differently. As with my friends Carol and David, there are always exceptions, lots of exceptions to how people in particular groups believe and behave.

Took a little Sabbath time for myself today with intervals of rest, "holy down time." Swam, ate tasty leftovers, and called family. After a late nap, I watched from my living room windows while the sunset colored a ribbon of sky crimson. Nature is holy.

Sunday, July 6, 2008

This morning went to our combined service where the preacher for the day was United Church of Christ minister, Michael Dowd. He held my attention from the first moment. For nearly an hour, I was flying among the planets and stars. The ideas in his book, *Thank God for Evolution* (Viking Penguin, New York, 2008), were riveting in the author's presentation.

Author Dowd and his scientist wife are itinerant; that is, they keep traveling and do not have a home of their own. They live as guests in their sponsor's houses, spending a rare night in a hotel. Constantly on the move, they continue to educate and inspire people in both religious and secular settings. Their mission is to promote a unique understanding of evolution as a natural marvel not in conflict with faith in God, but one that can expand our faith.

At the close of his sermon, Dowd said something like: "The two people who have contributed most to my journey are Jesus and Darwin," a statement which will either scare you, or thrill some to death. Today I found myself on the thrilling end.

I believe Michael Dowd's message is what the New Atheists and the religious fundamentalists need to hear, those at the opposite extremes of the faith continuum, as well as all of us in between: To care for ourselves and our planet we must not remain stuck in the habits of greed and profligate consumption. We must keep evolving.

Tuesday, July 22, 2008

Today I sat outside in a torrential rain, protected by the awning of our dormitory building at chaplains' retreat. The smell of rain beating down on grass has no match, nor does its sound of power and sweetness. Flying raindrops on my arms and face awakened and renewed my soul. Even Noah must have been moved at the start of God's big rain.

Tuesday, September 9, 2008

When mind and body are at peace, there's a natural rhythm to work and rest.

Wednesday, September 24, 2008

Read a Psalm and chapter from Ephesians while still in bed and passed a dreamy half hour putting in my eye drops. Unless I'm pressured to get out on the road, there are times when my preparations for the day are interrupted by spaces of meditation where I am simply present. Time is gone.

I told Monsignor John about these morning lapses. John was a retired priest I had met in an ecumenical clergy group during my first pastorate. We became friends. He was old and becoming frail. A few times I brought lunch to his little house way out in the country. He'd solemnly bless the food and table wine before we ate. One afternoon I confessed how, quite often, I would fall into this semi-conscious, time-wasting state, while pulling on my stockings in the morning. I'm not sure what feedback I expected. From my childhood on, family and friends have made fun of my absent-mindedness. The sin of "day-dreaming" was handwritten on my report card all through grade school.

"Sometimes," I confided to Monsignor John, "I have one leg in my stockings, and then I will be off in another world for a half hour before I remember to put in the other leg." This conversation was really about time and eternity.

He answered me with his trace of Irish brogue, his old eyes, kind: "That may be precious time," he said. "Think of this: When you stop, in the reverie, while you're so quiet, so still, you may have a chance to hear what the Lawd is sayin' to you."

Today, however, is a different story:

> "One stocking off an' one stocking on,
> an' I can't yet hear what the dear Lawd's sayin',
> Monsignor John."

The truth is, on remembering my old priest friend, my hearing improved.

Thursday, September 11, 2008

While driving I listened to music and commentary memorializing the people who died on 9/11. Images from that day return. On Tuesdays, area pastors still gather in the basement of the Lutheran church where we first heard the news. We have been meeting in that church for years to study together.

A little after 9:00 that day, we were sitting around the table, waiting for the rest of the group. The first late-arriving pastor told us about the first plane flying into the tower. The second pastor told us about the second plane. Stunned, we were unable to conceive the magnitude of the tragedy. For almost two hours we sat, at a loss to how we might address our congregations.

One of the hardest things to reconcile is the concept of a good God with the presence of evil in the world. Obviously, we must not reconcile with evil. We must acknowledge evil, take responsibility for some of it, try not to perpetuate it and, every day, ask God to deliver us from it.

Numerous prayer intentions in the United Methodist Worship Book begin with the phrase: "With God's help." I believe, with God's help, any person, in any condition can learn to do good in this world.

Tuesday, September 30, 2008

I'm singing in the ensemble for the High Holy Days this year. I love the service; there's so much music, the music of dancing, the music of longing. The rabbi spoke about hydration, not just hydration of the body, but hydration of the spirit, through *mitzvoth*, the good deeds we do for others. Glancing around the sanctuary, I wondered if the rabbi saw what I saw. Her words drew my attention to all those little bottles of spring water congregants held in their hands, or else propped up next to them in the pews, water bottles everywhere, leaning against handbags and prayer books, partially covered by prayer shawls. Such a hot night, though the air conditioning was on high, our thirst was cumulative. We singers had the best excuse for bottles on the floor near our chairs: our throats.

Next week, on Yom Kippur, not even water will be allowed. Tonight, the cantor left a bottle in plain sight, only yards from the Ark of the Covenant. The water, real and symbolic, became for me a kind of communion symbol. We were drinking together as well as singing and praying; we were taking God in. We were promising by our prayers, "with God's help," we would help people in need. There was real joy in the promise and expectation of joy in our voices.

No reason why the real Jesus could not be right there with us, singing the songs and sanctifying our intentions. Some of them were his songs, too. I think he would have been fine with the message and the company. I think, though, the Nazarene might be regarded as a troublemaker in this place, as he was in synagogues during his earthly life, and still is in many churches today.

Wednesday, October 8, 2008

These sacred songs carried me into the past. At service today I remembered two people I hurt years ago, and with whom I have not been able to reconcile.

Thursday, October 9, 2008

A Yom Kippur of silence, song, and holy readings. We sang from our 9:00 a.m. practice until almost 6:00 p.m. with an afternoon break of an hour and a half. My favorite time is the celebration of the Torah. The Scroll is handled by the faithful as though it were a human being, a child, really. There is the undressing, the taking off its glittering silver cap or crown, the blessing of and the cradling, then, the dancing. Men and women holding the Torah were dancing with the Scroll in their arms, the way we would with our own dear child; and all the while we sang together.

Back home, I began thinking about the representations of the holy family during the Christmas season. The crèche has become a kind of still life. Even live nativity scenes with real sheep and cows and, sometimes, a breathing flesh and blood baby "Jesus" compel us to stand at some distance. We cannot touch Him. There's singing, yes, but no one dances. Could we ever lift up the porcelain or olive-wood baby Jesus in our arms and dance with it around the sanctuary? I bet the shepherds danced.

Toward the end of the day, during the memorial service for those who had died during the past year, was the reading of a poem by Si Kahn. A woman from the congregation went to the podium, a lovely woman with fluffy brown hair, maybe a mother of children herself. She could not get through the reading, could barely speak after the first verse:

In the city of Warsaw such a long time ago
Two hundred children stand lined row on row
With their freshly washed faces and freshly washed clothes
The children of Poland who never grow old.

Another reader got up to take the young woman's place. Perhaps a grandmother, this time, I thought. Unlike the first woman, she was able to read without breaking down. A grandmother myself, feeling the tears wetting my cheeks, I wondered if mine were the tears she was holding back.

As our choir filed out one by one, a man decorated in a prayer shawl leaned over a pew and gathered me in his arms. "Thank you," he said, "thank you." Gratitude went both ways.

Healthy religion implies a preference for all that is life-giving, a belief in things unseen, and responsibility to a recognized community. In every case, members of these communities through the ages have been derided, denied, and murdered. The bond between God and the people is meant to hold the people together, yet must not keep them from including or protecting "the stranger."

Wednesday, November 12, 2008

Attended a soup supper at the reform synagogue where three women rabbis conducted a forum-type discussion advertised to address the theme of body and soul. They asked for questions. Finally, my unsigned query was pulled out of the box: "How can one perceive a person's soul from his or her mortal or bodily self?"

The youngest rabbi began by citing the *Midrash*. She told how in the rabbinic literature there are stories of angels appearing to reveal God's presence. She said once, when sitting with a dying person, she looked up and glimpsed an angel at the head of the bed. As she spoke, I could "see" that angel hovering around the headboard.

I've heard many such stories over the years. Yet, in ministering with the sick and dying, I've never spotted an identifiable angel. Only once, long ago, I saw what I imagined might be a group of "angels," which presented as a dizzying blur around a ceiling light. They spun above two dozen pastors singing our hearts out. This sighting happened during a Bible study retreat in Green Bay, Wisconsin.

Could the presence or perception of angelic entities be a sign of God's caring for a soul, as we *are* there, trying to do the same thing? The youngest rabbi went on to speak of the necessity of really looking at the person, of really listening, of being open, in order to be able see the Divine Spark.

The second rabbi referred to working with severely disabled persons, some who cannot care for themselves. She spoke also of seeing the Divine Spark in them. Henry Nouwen, renowned Jesuit author and priest, who devoted his later years to serving severely handicapped persons, spoke and wrote about recognizing the sacred *being* of each one he served.

For we who have SSc and other chronic diseases, caring for our bodies is important. We consult with various practitioners who may offer us medications and natural therapies. We search libraries and the Internet, hoping to discover ground-breaking possibilities for a cure. We write checks and/or give time to foundations and walk miles, or are wheeled, to help fund medical research.

Taking care of our souls is another story. Since caring for one's soul may distract us from coping with our disease, there must be a convincing argument for such dedication. The best reason I can offer is: All else may change, but our spiritual reality provides an enduring context for who we are.

When praying for someone during a service, I believe I'm in the company of the faithful, both those I see around me, and those I cannot see. In asking for the Light of Christ to surround and to fill the sick person, I have a sense of the gathering of the whole individual, body, mind, and spirit, within that protective, transforming circle of Light.

All the world's major religions have a heaven. Judaism contains many references to everlasting life. To me, the most appealing of these is the joy of studying Torah in eternity with Father Abraham, perhaps because I've experienced the joy of studying Torah on earth with some wise teachers, among them a few women, or "Mother Sarahs," as I have called them.

I've been thinking about how belief in eternal life might impact the lives we are living here and now. Belief in eternal life may keep a person from giving up hope, no matter what the circumstance, simply from implication of continuance. I have had several life experiences leading to my conviction that Love is stronger than death; this is the Love which carries us forth. I would be happy to live here as long as I can, leaning into every moment. When my time comes, I hope I will be as happy to go, and even happier to arrive where the ancestral saints reside, and those intractable angels sing.

Sunday, December 28, 2008

Felt an inner emptiness this morning, a hunger for the Bread of Heaven. Stopped off early at my old home church where the book group meets, but they were having holiday recess. Unwilling to wait an hour for the service, I drove to the church where I'll be guest preacher next week. The story was Simeon's receiving Jesus on the day his parents brought him to the temple for the ritual circumcision. Old Simeon sees deeply into the being of the Infant, proclaiming he is free to die now that his ultimate longing to see the Lord has been fulfilled. He asks the Infant's blessing.

The pastor brought the message home, about Simeon's recognizing the wisdom of the Messiah in the baby's face, and how our hearing or knowing is not enough. We ourselves must look deeply and long to see his wisdom. For us to say: "Hail Mary, full of grace," also is not enough. We ourselves need to come closer to God, so we, like Mary, may be filled with Grace.

Wednesday, January 28, 2009

Yesterday, waiting for a client, I re-read the opening page of Thomas R Kelly's *A Testament of Devotion* (1941, Harper, San Francisco, 1996), a slim volume containing thoughts on meditation and the practice of prayer. The first sentence is a quote from Meister Eckhart, German theologian and writer (1260-1328).

"As thou art, in church or cell, that same frame of mind carry out into the world, into its turmoil, and its fitfulness." Thomas Kelly speaks again from his own heart: "Deep within us all there is an amazing inner sanctuary of the soul, a holy place, a Divine Center, a speaking Voice, to which we may continuously return."

Reflecting, journaling, counseling, saying hello to a stranger in the elevator, driving in heavy traffic, sitting with my closest friend—these moments are enhanced when I do not venture too far from that place within. How do I stay true to the Path even when I do not know where it is taking me? The practice of inner quiet and devotion, I believe, increases awareness of God's presence and is central to the healing process.

Saturday, January 31, 2009

After reading two verses of Psalm 127, I memorized them. As a child, memorizing was the magical way I could "hear" a poem or verse whenever I wished. In graduate school, when reading an assigned book in its entirety was more than I could manage, I scanned each chapter, took notes, and memorized key passages. This not only helped in taking essay examinations, I still can whisper my favorite poems in the darkness. Blake, Yeats, Dickenson, and St. Vincent Millay are among my favorites. My Psalm of the night:

> *Unless the Lord builds a house,*
> *those who build it labor in vain.*
> *Unless the Lord guards the city,*
> *the guard keeps watch in vain.*
> *It is in vain that you rise up early*
> *and go late to rest,*
> *eating the bread of anxious toil;*
> *for he gives sleep to his beloved.*
> *~Psalm 127: 1-2 (NRSV)*

I need Help building everything I put my hands to. After a long day, when we slow down, the Eternal One who watches over the city promises to watch over us. No need to worry, or to be hypervigilant; "for he gives sleep to his beloved."

Wednesday, February 4, 2009

This week my soul rebelled. More convincing than the evils of mere physical or psychological stress is when the soul itself calls us to task, when the soul says: "stop."

Saturday, February 7, 2009

While applying castor oil to my body, I remembered something I learned while staying at a Benedictine retreat house in Bethesda a decade ago. I can pray an intention to dedicate my day to someone in pain or trouble or to some place where people are in great need. Dedication of a day is an invisible and wordless act no one else has to know about. Essentially, I place myself in solidarity with some especially fragile soul or territory.

Still applying the castor oil, I recalled how Edgar Cayce reminds us of the importance of being conscious of the Source of healing. Simply following a prescribed action is not enough and, like an uninspired ritual, has little good to offer.

In Cayce's words:

"Do not make the applications merely as routine, either the rubs, the diets, or the appliance. Let these be done with the continuous spiritual purpose to be healed of the disturbances FOR a definite purpose, that is to be constructive and helpful to others...Keep optimistic. Pray often; seeing, feeling, asking, desiring, expecting help—from Him, who is the way, the truth, and the light."

(Edgar Cayce, A.R.E., from *Circulating File on Scleroderma*)

Sunday, February 22, 2009

My massage therapist brought me to a state of complete painlessness that lasted through yesterday and overnight. No pain when I got up this morning. Joints and muscles quiet. For a while, I had no desire to accomplish a thing. My only wish was to preserve this almost weightless state as long as possible.

An hour of working on the apartment, an hour at the computer and, naturally, the old tension's beginning to accumulate in my back and neck. Pain's on the way to rejoining me. However, yesterday's body massage has changed understanding of pain and pleasure. Pain can be motivation for change, while pleasure is a lovely resting place. Pain is contraction. Pleasure is expansion. This dynamic is the rule even of our heart muscle and underlies every worthy effort:

contract, expand; contract, expand. My journey to healing includes the submission of both pain and pleasure to God. The inner balance I desire cannot be attained entirely through my own efforts.

Tuesday, March 3, 2009

Shamelessly asking my friends to pray for tomorrow's procedure. I've asked by email, telephone, and in person. Trying to make the task easy for them, I say, "Send one up for me, would you?" trusting God will forgive the casual language I use to disguise my urgent request.

One of my swim buddies is a parish visitor and liturgist in her church. With her, I was straightforward about my concerns. She made a commitment to pray for me during the entire endoscope procedure as did another friend who attends Wednesday-morning Eucharist.

This Lent, I'm trying to be more caring of myself. Although, the Church sanctifies men and women for reportedly loving others better than themselves, I have serious doubts about whether such total self-denying love is possible. A poem by William Blake describes the impossibility of loving another "better" than oneself:

> *Naught loves another as itself*
> *Nor venerates another so,*
> *Nor is it possible to Thought*
> *A greater than itself to know.*
> *So Father, how can I love you,*
> *Or any of my brothers more?*
> *I love you as I love the bird*
> *That picks up crumbs around the door.*

~William Blake, "A Little Boy Lost"

The boy in the poem speaks honestly of loving those he sees who are close to him; he loves the "bird" with the same love with which he loves the Father, or his brothers. In later verses, the boy is seized by the hair, and taken to a "holy place" to be burned by priests for his sin of heresy. This is a fine example of how religion can get sick to death, even violent, when controlling takes the place of loving.

"Little Boy Lost" is a good lesson for compulsive caretakers, for people who may be struggling to fulfill others' expectations of them, people like us, with diseases like scleroderma. Often, driven by guilt or misguided altruism, we sometimes offer more than we have to give. The child in Blake's poem admits his limitations in loving as naturally and honestly as he can. We might admit our own limitations, as honestly, if only we could.

Tuesday, March 10, 2009

Was up before dawn, feeling much better. I recognize my need to be spiritually centered for my own sake as well as the sake of every one in my system. Bringing this intention to my yoga stretches, cleaning up the kitchen, medication-taking, an hour-long breakfast, and my plan for the day.

Friday, March 13, 2009

Bob's left to go home. I'm sitting alone at the dining room table, looking out at the tower of St. Patrick's cathedral, beautiful in every season, especially on this cold, sunny March afternoon. Close by my plate is a cut-glass pitcher with purple columbine, a Lenten flower. My whole body is longing to absorb the loveliness around me. In my growing hunger for food and life, I want swallow up all that beauty coming in too slowly through my pores.

Wednesday, March 19, 2009

Got up early for the service with laying on of hands. A small group of regulars, deacons, pastors, and other people meet for this half hour on Wednesday mornings. We consider a Psalm together and pray for those who are sick, take communion, and wait for the sign of the cross to be drawn on our foreheads with oil. Over the past seventeen years I've often been the pastor designated to serve and do the anointing blessing.

Toward the close, a chair is placed in the center of the circle for anyone who wishes to receive the laying on of hands. Today, the called pastor sat in the chair first; I was next. Asked my friend Ellie to put her hand directly over the ulcer site; didn't think she'd have a problem touching me between breast and belly. The others put their hands on my shoulders, head, and back. In those moments of prayer, through the very warmth of their hands, I could feel Christ's healing Love.

Wednesday, April 29, 2009

Realized this afternoon, walking over the mountaintop of the monastery's farmland, how much I've missed intimacy with trees. Ever since childhood, trees have had a way of moving me toward gentleness, toward peace. Last night, from my window, I watched their branches swaying in the wind and rain. In today's late afternoon sunshine they were reaching toward me with a softer motion, as though inviting me to restore our life-long friendship.

A Final Word

For those willing to go to the trouble to make the changes appropriate to their needs, particularly with regard to nutrition and exercise, improvement in physical health is possible at almost any stage of SSc. Expectations of a good result and trust in one's healing network, as well as keeping a daily record of progress and setbacks, will help to bring this about.

If you are a patient, teach your caregivers. If you are a health professional, learn from your patients. As you are able, acknowledge the working of an invisible Power. All of these, with a balanced collaboration between patient and clinician, hold the greatest promise for optimal health.

GLOSSARY

ACE inhibitors. **A family of drugs used to treat systemic hypertension (and malignant hypertension of scleroderma renal crisis).**

Acid Reflux. Splashing up of stomach acid into esophagus and throat.

ALD. Schilder's disease, rare and usually fatal within ten years of onset.

Alkalinity. Opposite of acidity.

Allergy. Body reaction to substances or situations affecting a minority of people, i.e. sneezing, rashes, respiratory distress.

Alveoli. Tiny airs sac in lungs.

ANA. Antinuclear antibody; antibodies that attack nuclear contents of body cells.

Anemia. Insufficient red blood cells.

Antibodies. Proteins the body produces to reject infections or other unwanted invaders.

Anti-centromere. An antibody that targets a portion of the chromosomes of the nucleus of cells most commonly found in persons with the limited form scleroderma.

Anti-Scl70 antibody. An antinuclear antibody that targets a portion of the chromosomes of the nucleus of cells most commonly found in persons with the diffuse form of scleroderma.

Arrhythmia. Irregular heartbeat or rhythm.

Aspiration. The inadvertent inhalation of food or liquid.

Atrium. Either left or right heart chamber into which veins pour blood.

Atrophy. Wasting of muscle or other tissue.

Autoimmune disease. Condition in which immune system attacks one's own body cells.

Autonomic nervous system. Regulates unconscious working of gastrointestinal, respiratory, heart, and other internal body organ functions, falls into sympathetic and parasympathetic categories.

Barrett's Syndrome. Pre-cancerous cells in esophageal lining near the stomach.

Bell's Palsy. Nerve damage, where part or all of one side of the face is paralyzed.

Biopsy. A procedure to remove tissue or cells for microscopic evaluation.

Calcinosis. Calcium salt deposits under or at surface of the skin.

Capillaries. Smallest blood vessels.

Castor Oil Pack Directions. A cloth, ideally of unbleached wool or cotton flannel, folded in three or four layers of thickness and able to well cover the area for healing, is moistened with cold-pressed castor oil, and then placed over the area. Thin plastic wrap may be stretched over the cloth and wrapped around the limb or body to hold the pack in place, and protect one's surrounding clothing or bedding from oil leakage. A heating pad or hot water bottle is then held over area for continued warmth for an hour or more depending on the ailment being treated. After pack is removed, a washcloth dipped in warm baking soda and water will effectively clean off any toxins that have come to the surface. The pack may be applied for four days or nights in a row, and then skipped a day, before continuing applications for the next four days or until symptoms subside. Edgar Cayce recommends a time of prayer and meditation be observed during these applications. All ingredients and items can be purchased individually from health food and fabric stores, or the Castor Oil Pack Kit can be ordered from the Baar catalog, 1-800-269-2502, or online at www.baar.com.

CHF. Congestive heart failure.

Collagen. A connective tissue protein that makes up the majority of skin tissue, and is important in the formation and holding together of all body structures and organ linings.

Contracture. Permanent shortening of muscle or tendon.

Cranial neuropathy. Nerve damage to the brain.

C.R.E.S.T. Acronym now mostly out of use; referring to five symptoms of the systemic forms of scleroderma: calcinosis, Raynaud's syndrome, esophageal dysfunction, sclerodactyly, and telangiectasia.

Diffuse. Affecting a greater area of the body, as in organs or multiple systems.

Digital ulcers. Open sores on fingers and toes, a result of cellular damage from Raynaud's.

Dismotility. When esophageal, or other areas of intestinal walls do not contract normally in order to keep ingested food moving downward.

Edema. Water retention in tissues, causing swelling.

En coup de saber. Occurs in localized scleroderma; presents as scarred line on head, face, scalp or neck; French for "cut from a sword."

Endoscopy, or endoscope procedure. Small instruments are swallowed or inserted into the rectum for examination, biopsy, or onsite treatment of digestive tract.

Esophageal dysfunction. Impaired flow downward of food from mouth to stomach.

Fibrosis. Hardened tissue that may interfere with bodily functions.

Gastrointestinal Reflux. *See* acid reflux, or GERD.

Genetics. Study of relationship of disease to family health history.

GERD. Gastroesophageal reflux disease.

GI Tract. Gastrointestinal passage from mouth to anus.

Hemoglobin A1C. Blood test that reveals three month average of blood sugar levels.

Hypertension. Elevated blood pressure.

H2 blockers. Drugs to block or neutralize stomach acid.

IBS. See Irritable bowel syndrome.

Immune system. System of biological processes designed to protect body against disease.

Irritable bowel syndrome. May include bouts of diarrhea, constipation, and abdominal pain.

Ligament. Bands of tissue connecting bones to one another.

Limited scleroderma. Type less likely to cause early onset of organ damage, characterized primarily by Raynaud's and esophageal dysfunction.

Linear scleroderma. Type characterized by line of scarred tissue, usually one face or head.

Localized scleroderma. Form restricted to specific area of the body.

Lupus. (systemic lupus erythematosus) A chronic autoimmune disease characterized by pain and inflammation, may affect spinal cord, brain, skin and internal organs.

Malabsorption. Condition where the body cannot effectively utilize nutrients and calories from food.

Morphea. Irregular patches of thickened skin.

Multiple sclerosis (MS). A neurological inflammatory disease that affects brain and spinal cord, in which the patient's immune system attacks the nerves.

Mucus membrane. Naturally moist areas of the body, such as mouth.

MS. See multiple sclerosis.

Myopathy. Pertaining to muscle pain or dysfunction.

Neuron. Nerve cell.

Neuropathy. Portion of the body affected by nerve damage, numbness.

Orphan disease. Referring to scleroderma as a minority, or rare disease.

Osteoporosis. Rheumatic condition, often post-menopausal, where bones become porous and more easily breakable.

Oximeter. Oxygen measuring device usually clipped to finger or earlobe during tests and procedures.

PAH. *See* pulmonary arterial hypertension.

Pericarditis. Inflamed lining around the heart.

PPI. *See* proton-pump inhibitor.

Probiotics. Bacteria friendly to the intestines, found in certain cultured milk and yogurt products.

Proton pump inhibitor. A type of drug that inhibits production of stomach acid.

Pulmonary. Involving the lungs.

Pulmonary Arterial Hypertension. Increased pressure within lung arteries, causing high blood pressure.

Raynaud's Phenomena. Condition where fingers and toes turn red, white, and then blue in reaction to cold or stress.

Reflux. Splashing up of stomach acid into the mouth.

Remission. Temporary or permanent cessation of illness.

Renal. Pertaining to kidneys.

Renin. Protein made by kidneys.

Scleroderma. Autoimmune connective tissue disease.

Sclerosis. Disease involving hardening of body tissue.

Sjogren's Syndrome. Condition where mucus membranes become extremely dry.

Sphincter. Muscular "door" that keeps food from traveling up through esophagus and waste from leaking from anus.

SSc. Systemic forms of systemic sclerosis or scleroderma.

Steroids. Drugs that temporarily increase muscle strength and function.

Stricture. Narrowing.

Syndrome. Group of symptoms relating to particular condition.

Systemic. Affecting much of the body.

Systemic Lupus Erythematosus. *See* lupus.

Systemic sclerosis. Another term for scleroderma, indicating both its broad effect on body systems and tissue hardening.

Telangiecgasias. Blood vessels that expand and break close to surface of skin or mucus membranes in mouth, causing red spots.

Tendon rub. Audible sound made by tendon rubbing against tendon sheath.

Ulcers. Sores or focused areas of inflammation, which may bleed.

Vascular. Pertaining to blood vessels.

Venous. Pertaining to veins.

Watermelon stomach. (gastric antral vascular ectasia) A condition where stomach lining appears striped from dilated blood vessels, which may bleed.

ACKNOWLEDGEMENTS

My thanks to the staff of the Scleroderma Foundation's Tri-State Chapter who has been a wonderful resource, lending me books and CDs, and answering my many questions. Also, thanks to my friends and family, co-op neighbors, colleagues, and health practitioners who generously encouraged this project.

Special thanks to Ruth R. Bass, Nathalie Caminiti, Sybil Goldenberg, Barbara Alhart Simon, and Norman K. Sloan, for reading and providing feedback on my first drafts; to Ruth, who said, "Even persons without scleroderma could benefit"; to Nathalie who spent precious vacation time reading aloud with me; to Sybil, who, over winter cups of tea, encouraged a more conversational style; to Barbara, who called me to better organization; and to Norman for his helpful red markings and editorial advice.

Thank you to my editor, Marly Cornell, whose skill and guidance have been invaluable to me.

The three persons with whom I was in closest communication are Diane Tolentino, Robert J. Armitage, and my scleroderma specialist, Dr. Lee S. Shapiro. Diane kept the manuscript up to date by monitoring backups, and came speedily to the rescue when my computers played tricks on me. Thank you, Diane! Heartfelt thanks to my dear friend Bob who provided stellar support and was nearly always available to talk or listen. I owe my deepest gratitude to Dr. Shapiro who read the early drafts, corrected my medical prose; and sent me feedback over a period of two years, while caring for his patients and working on research and writing of his own.

ABOUT THE AUTHOR

Bianca Podesta was born in Northern New Jersey, where she grew up dreaming of becoming a singer or writer. She earned degrees in music and English from Centenary College and Columbia University. As a mother with a young child, she was discouraged from pursuing her interest in medicine because she lacked science credits and financial backing. Podesta received a doctorate in psychology in 1975 from Union Institute (UGS) and worked as a counselor in New York and New Jersey before going to Drew Theological School where she earned her Master of Divinity. After being ordained a United Methodist minister, she served a number of churches before being certified as a pastoral counselor. She is a Fellow in the American Association of Pastoral Counselors. In 2001 she completed the program in Spiritual Direction at Shalem Institute. Currently she works as counselor and spiritual director with a non-profit counseling ministry in upstate New York. She has a son and two grandchildren, and sings with The Madrigal Choir of Binghamton.